Lady's Companion For

PMS

Treated Naturally

Mark Gilberd
Homoeopath. Medical Herbalist and Iridologist

Index

(Siberian), Ginger, Hops Hops, Ladys Mantle, Maca,Milk Thistle, Motherwort, Passion Flower, Raspberry, Red Clover, Rosemary, Sage, St Johns Wort, Schizandra, Sarsaparilla, Shepherds Purse, Skullcap, Squaw Vine, Valerian, Vervain, Vitex (Chaste Tree), Yarrow, Wild Yam, Withania, Zizyphus.

Homoeopathic Supplement

Symptom Questions Guide
Treatment Using The Kit
The Four Complexes
How To Take The Complexes
Example Of A Dose
How To Use This Section

Materia Medica (Homoeopathic Remedies List)

Aconite, Allium Cepa, Antimonium Tartaricum, Apis, Arnica, Arsenic Album,Belladonna, Bellis Perennis, Bryonia, Calendula,Cantharis, Carbo Vegetabilis,Causticum, Cimicfuga,Euphrasia, Hypericum,Ignatia,Ipecac, Kali Bichromicum, Kali Carbonicum, Lachesis,Ledum,Lycopodium, Natrum Sulphuricum,Nux Vom, Phosphorus, Pulsatilla,Rhus Tox, Ruta, Silica, Staphysagria

,Sepia, Symphytum, Tarentula Cubensis, Urtica Urens

Introduction

I wrote this over a decade ago but now here the laws have changed and I am not allowed to prescribe without seeing the patient so I have had to change this from being a Kit with medicine supplied to just giving you the recipe of the remedies used in the Kit. The Kit was designed originally for people in remote areas in outback Australia where there can be little help for the day to day problems and specialists only pop up every six months if you are lucky. It was designed to empower the patient and give simple and safe treatment using Homoeopathic Remedies whose formula I kept secret but will now give to the world. I have always been upset by the way our modern medical system seeks to disempower you and leave you stranded and dependent on them. In the decade gone they have not made any real insights into PMS and there doesn't seem to be anything coming up. I will now let you read the old Foreword and original add for the kit.

Regards

Mark Gilberd

Foreword

This booklet and kit has been designed and made for practical people who are not afraid to take their own fate in their hands and do something about it. The booklet is set out in such a way as to empower you and put the control of your health back into your hands where it belongs. Too many people in this life just sit back and do what their Doctor tells them whether they like it or not and leave it up to fate to decide their future, it is a bit like pointing the bone especially if you say the cancer word. The reality is if you have been on a junk food diet all your life and spend 30 hours or more in front of the TV a week your chances of getting healthy again regardless how much medication you take are very slim.

This booklet gives you information about PMS and introduces you to the common symptoms and gives you a way of recording your own personal symptoms in a way that will show up any type of pattern that might be happening. Latter we go into diet and show how this can affect some of the symptoms and health in general and then we move on to supplements that can be taken which work to increase your health and relieve your problems.

Next we move on to how to use the Homoeopathic Complexes which are the medication supplied with the Kit that can be mixed together in such a way as to cover your own personal symptoms.

If after this you are still having problems then you could move onto Herbal treatment which can be very effective but the most important thing is that by then you would of done most of the ground work yourself. For example your nutrition would have improved, you would also be taking the correct nutritional supplements for your condition, you would also have your own symptom chart which would probably be showing a pattern by now so you would have covered a lot of ground and be well on the way to a healthier future.

Last of all I want to say especially to people with severe problems don't be afraid of using Hormone Treatment that Doctors usually prescribe for severe problems as this form of treatment can bring reasonably fast relief and you can use this treatment to get yourself over the worst of the problems then slowly wean yourself off as your health improves. Problems with hormone replacement therapy seem only to happen to the long time users but if you use it just to get yourself over the worst and improve your health while you are doing this and keep on using your chart you should come out alright at the end.

Well best of luck

Mark Gilberd

Homoeopath, Medical Herbalist and Iridologist.

Accredited With The Australian Traditional Medicine Society

The PMS Kit

This is a unique product designed for women who live in remote areas and who have to travel great distances to see a Doctor. It gives all the information you need on how to attack the problem symptoms and a system of recording your own personal symptoms (Symptom Diary) which will help to show you the future problems you may expect and is a valuable record for a Doctors future reference. The Kit contains a Booklet giving you all the information you need with a plan on how to attack the problem and even how to predict the future!. Once you've predicted the future (through your Symptom Diary) you can now attack the symptoms before they even begin. The Kit contains a Booklet giving you the information you need with sections on Causes, The Common Symptoms of PMS, Symptoms In Detail with Supplements and Herb Lists, Diet and Nutrition, Common Supplements and at the back of the booklet there is a Comprehensive Herbal with 40 Female suitable herbs, a list of 38 different Herbal Actions along with the Herbs and lots more. The second to last page is devoted to the use of the Homoeopathic Complexes that are a part of the kit and it teaches you how to use them to match your personal symptoms.

The Kit comes with 4 Homoeopathic Complexes that work like this.
There are 4 Stock Bottles in the kit and they are labeled

PMS(A). This complex has the two hormones estrogen and progesterone in it. I have made it in such a way that it will reduce the strength of estrogen and encourage more production of progesterone. The other 4 remedies I have in this complex will help to counter the symptoms of **Anxiety, Irritability, Mood Swings** and **Nervous Tension**.

PMS(B) Mixer. In this complex there are no hormones so you can safely mix it with another. There are 4 remedies in this complex and they will help to counter the symptoms of **Fluid Retention, Weight Gain, Breast Tenderness, Abdominal Tenderness, Swollen Hands and Feet**. This complex mixes well with PMS(A) as PMS(A) has the low estrogen hormone in it and high estrogen is part of the cause for bloating.

PMS(C) Mixer. In this complex there are no hormones so you can safely mix it with another. There are 4 remedies in this complex and they will help to counter the symptoms of **Food Cravings, Headache, Fatigue, Dizziness and Palpitation.**

PMS(D). This complex has the hormones estrogen and progesterone in it. The complex will encourage estrogen production and reduce the production of progesterone this is the opposite of PMS(A) so for obvious reasons do no mix with PMS(A). The other 4 remedies in this complex cover the symptoms of **Depression, Crying, Forgetfulness, Confusion and Insomnia.**

The Kit also has a separate Acid and Alkaline Chart and Nutrition Guide.

The chart allows you to see if your body may be excessively acid. If this is the case your body may be stealing minerals from your bones or anywhere it can to make the body more alkaline especially the blood and in turn this could lead to osteoporosis. Excessively acid bodies may lead to arthritis and other disease conditions. The nutrition section includes Nutrition For The Reproductive System and an introduction to the herb Maca which slowly over time may rejuvenate the endocrine system and balance all the hormone systems of the body.

Feel better and take control of your life today.

The Modern Medical Approach

The 3 Step Approach

Step 1: Mild To Moderate Symptoms - Many Doctors adopt a step wise approach to treating PMS with the first step being to establish if it is PMS. After this they may give advice on lifestyle such as a healthy diet, exercise, relaxation or stress management and other ways you can begin to modify your lifestyle. They may suggest some simple over the counter remedies or supplements or write you a prescription for a simple diuretic (water tablet) or a mild supplement such as evening Primrose oil to alleviate breast tenderness. They may also suggest you visit a Women's Health Clinic or may refer you for counseling if psychological symptoms are troublesome.

If the symptoms don't go or get worse after about 2 to 3 months you will probably move on to Step 2.

Step 2: Moderate To Severe Symptoms - The precise treatments vary but may include prescription medications for the treatment of breast tenderness and other symptoms, Hormonal treatments such as progesterone for physical and mental symptoms, the contraceptive pill so as to stop ovulation (PMS symptoms begin after ovulation) and control hormonal levels or maybe estrogen patches. Antidepressants of the SSRI Group (SSRI means selective serotonin reuptake inhibitors a common one is Prozac) could be given for psychological symptoms such as mood swing, depression and sugar cravings. If you don't respond to Step 2 you will move up to Step 3.

Step 3: Severe Symptoms - This involves usually referring you to a Specialist a Gynaecologist or sometimes a psychiatrist who may prescribe medication for around 6 months which suppress the hormones that trigger ovulation. In effect this triggers an artificial menopause. For this reason the Doctor may also prescribe other drugs such as Hormone Replacement Therapy (HRT) to prevent menopausal symptoms and to protect your bones. In rare and extreme instances if all else fails the Specialist may recommend a Hysterectomy with removal of the ovaries. In this case you will be offered HRT to prevent Menopausal Symptoms and to protect your bones.

The Common Symptoms of PMS

1/. Feelings of depression, sadness, pessimism.

2/. Tiredness, lethargy, feelings of being under the weather.

3/. Tension, irritability, anxiety.

4/. Increased or decreased appetite.

5/. Cravings for sweet or salty food.

6/. Thirst.

7/. Lack of concentration, difficulties in decision making.

8/. Weepiness.

9/. Mood swings.

10/. Feeling extra sexy or losing interest in sex.

11/. Inability to sleep or wanting to sleep all the time.

12/. Aggressive outbursts, impulsive behavior.

13/. Increased energy

14/. Loss of confidence and self-esteem, wanting to stay indoors all the time.

15/. Guilt feelings, putting yourself down.

16/. Loss of interest in yourself.

17/. Apathy

18/. Headache or migraine.

19/. Breast swelling and tenderness.

20/. Bloating or feeling of bloatedness.

21/. Swollen fingers and toes.

22/. Acne, rashes, itching.

23/. Constipation, nausea, diarrhea.

24/. Poor coordination. Clumsiness, becoming accident prone.

25/. Muscle weakness, backache, muscle pain.

26/. Dizziness.

27/. Weight Gain.

28/. Increased sweatiness.

29/. Blurred vision, sore eyes.

30/. Passing an increased or decreased amount of urine.

31/. Increased vaginal discharge.

32/. Pain in lower abdomen.

33/. Decreased efficiency

Notes

What Next

If you have answered yes to a lot of the above then you probably have a problem that you would like to do something about. PMS is one of the hardest conditions to treat. After well over a decade it is still hard for me to treat it but I know what to do now to clear the confusion. When I first started it was so hard to determine the most important symptoms to prescribe on as there were so many and usually the patient had a hard time to determine which was worse than the other and we would lead each other into more confusion. I started to think, this really is a battle and I am not doing well, maybe it's a battle I can't win. After dwelling on it for a while I decided if it is a battle I will treat it as a battle. So how do the military treat battles. The first thoughts were with discipline and intelligence. Discipline told me that there was no quick fix so you're going to have to be in it for the long haul. Intelligence told me that you could not beat an enemy until you knew how it works. So after deciding that there was no quick fix the obvious way of gathering intel on the enemy was to make the patients keep a Menstrual Diary listing all the different symptoms as they happen at the time they happened. Of course I would deal with any main symptoms that bothered the patient but I tried to do this in a gentle way so as not to cloud the picture of the main cause. After 3 months of using the Menstrual Diary there usually emerged a pattern that stood out and was obvious. I used to make a comment when looking at the diary that someone was pulling your strings and sometimes someone was even yanking your strings. When you see it plainly in front you it becomes obvious to you what to do and for the patient it is a great relief as they can see that they are not going crazy, there is something that's happening to Them that's following a pattern so that now they have a chance to predict the future and arrange their life accordingly.

After gathering all the intelligence it's time to see just who our enemy really is and how strong their positions are. After we have gotten to know them it is time to plan the attack. Nutrition is where you always start first. Next is to try the Homoeopathic Complexes to try to get the appropriate hormones under control and then to gauge the results after we have established which form of PMS you have or which one is the worst. For example PMS-A,B, C or D as the hormones will be going different ways for each of them which is one of the main important reasons to keep the Menstrual Calendar so as to distinguish which type of PMS it is. Latter if we get no good results from the complexes we move on to the herbs but hopefully before we get to the herbs nutrition has already been sorted out and is giving some help.

PMS Risk Factors And Causes

1/. Family History - There seems to be a genetic association so if someone in the family has got it then you may get it as well.

2/. A Hormonal Trigger Can Cause Or Increase The Severity Of PMS - e.g. the onset of puberty and menses, after pregnancy especially when there has been complications, postnatal depression, miscarriage, starting the pill though the onset of symptoms here can be very gradual and easy to miss so that it is only when the pill is stopped that the pattern is noticed and maybe a year or two before menopause can trigger PMS. Sterilization is another common starting point for PMS.

3/. Stress - PMS may appear after a long period of stress maybe from relationships or from financial problems or other life problems. New studies show that this might happen by a raise in the levels of one of the stress hormones called cortisol produced by the adrenal glands and is involved in triggering irritability and anger. Cortisol competes with progesterone for receptors that enable progesterone to enter the cells of the body, so if your stress levels are high you may end up with symptoms of progesterone deficiency.

4/. Increasing Age - PMS typically worsens during the 30s peaking in the mid to late 30s. During the 40s the symptoms start mixing with the menopause symptoms.

5/. Poor Nutrition - Sometimes a change to a good and healthy diet solves the problem.

6/. Alcohol - Many PMS sufferers have difficulty in coping with alcohol, especially Red Wine. In the good times they can have their daily triple without any problem but during their final premenstrual days they may find that they become intoxicated by an amount that would not normally bother them. What is worse they tend to have a great urge for more alcohol at these times.

7/. Tendency To Food Cravings And Binges - A very high proportion of PMS sufferers have difficulty in controlling their craving and binges usually for chocolates, sweets, starchy and even salty foods.

8/. Increased Sexual Urge - Young Teenagers and women as well may find they have an increased sex urge premenstrual.

9/. Symptom Magnification - PMS can make the pains of other conditions worse e.g. Arthritis.

10/. Hypothyroidism - Severe PMS can occur as a result of Hypothyroidism.

Do any of the above event relate to you if so which ones?

Notes

Factors Which Cause PMS To Increase In Severity

1/. Stress

2/. Night Work

3/. Large weight gain or loss.

4/. Poor Diet

5/. Smoking.

6/. Alcohol

Know Your Enemy

It is after ovulation that the main problems begin with PMS. In a women without PMS the levels estrogen to progesterone remain in sufficient and balanced amounts between ovulation and menstrual bleeding. In women with PMS the levels of estrogen and progesterone are out of balance. Researchers have found that women who have to low estrogen compared to progesterone complain of depression during the premenstrual phase. There can be many different variations in the hormone strengths creating many different combinations of symptoms and problems.

How Should It Be Diagnosed

In PMS the symptoms or complaints come only before menstruation and disappear after menstruation. Furthermore the complaints cannot start earlier then

14 days before menstruation. The same problems come each month at about the same phase in each menstrual cycle with monotonous regularity. Experts have recently identified 4 distinct patterns of PMS related to the time of the monthly cycle at which they are experienced.

Pattern 1/. Symptoms begin during the week before your period and recede during your period.

Pattern 2/. Symptoms start around the time of ovulation and persist until your period starts - that is for about 2 weeks.

Pattern 3/. A brief spell of symptoms are experienced around ovulation and then goes away, symptoms recur during the week before menstruation. This pattern often affects teenagers.

Pattern 4/. Symptoms come on around ovulation and continue over the next weeks and right through menstruation leaving just a week or 10 days without symptoms.

Whether these patterns relate to an underlying cause is not yet known but they may be useful in identifying days or weeks when PMS is more likely to be troublesome and may allow you to take steps to adjust your lifestyle.

Keeping A Menstrual Calendar Is The Best Way To Diagnose PMS.

Phases Of The Menstrual Cycle

Phase One Menstruation – Days 1 to 5

The hypothalamus part of the brain sends FSH (follicle stimulating hormone) to the pituitary gland known as the master gland or the conductor of the hormone orchestra, located also in the brain between the eyes and down a little bit. The pituitary then sends FSH to the ovaries to get the next egg ready.

Phase Two Proliferative Stage – 1 to 12

The egg cell begins to develop into a fluid filled follicle and grows enough to force itself to the surface of the ovary where it forms a sort of bubble. As the follicle develops it secretes estrogen adding to the quantity already being produced by the ovaries. The rise in the estrogen signals the womb and stimulates the lining to begin to grow.

Phase Three Ovulation - 13 to 15

When estrogen is 6 times higher than its starting level about 13 days after the onset of menstruation it signals the pituitary gland to drop the levels of FSH and to stimulate the release of LH (Luteinizing Hormone) which is the signal for the follicle to release the egg.

Phase Four The Luteal Phase – 16 to 28

The egg now enters the tube to begin the journey to the womb and under the influence of LH turns yellow and is now known as the Corpus Luteum and starts producing progesterone as well as estrogen. Progesterone thickens the lining of the womb and prepares the womb for the possibility of fertilization.

Phase Five Premenstrual

If the egg is not fertilized it shrinks and fades away and the supply of progesterone is shut off and the level of estrogen drops down. The lining of the womb begins to contract cutting the blood supplies and begins to shed causing the womb to contract and expel the debris causing menstruation. Then the cycle begins again.

What Are Hormones

The word hormone comes from the Greek word horman, which means to stir up, or arouse to activity. This is a good description for it is exactly what hormones do. Hormones are made in small glands throughout the body and from there use the blood circulation to travel to their destination. Each one has a specific job to do on its target organ or tissue, usually controlling, activating or directing certain functions. Many hormones can have an effect on your urges, desires, feelings and emotions just by the different strengths and mixtures that they are working at. Fluctuating hormone levels will vary throughout your life but there main fluctuating moments will be in Adolescence and Menopause which you could say is the reverse of Adolescence.

Hormones when you are young trigger your growth spurts especially at puberty, then throughout your life they control the speed of your metabolism at one extreme maybe making you a skinny high speed workaholic while at the other extreme a slow individual who is prone to putting on weight. Hormones balance your blood sugar and also have an effect on your bodies water balance along with affecting your breathing and the nervous system. To a certain degree hormones rule so we have to be very careful before we start playing around with this complex system.

As mentioned before some women can live their whole life and have no problems with this system while others have known nothing but problems. Hormonal upsets can arise from the use of the birth control pill or other hormone containing medicines or more natural conditions such as pregnancy or from a miscarriage. Surgery and operations such as hysterectomy or sterilization or even violence and mental trauma can throw the hormone system out of whack and lead on to many unwanted and annoying symptoms. Stress, lifestyle and genetic inheritance are major factors in hormone problems with each needing an investigation if problems are arising, sometimes it can be as simple as just changing your lifestyle while at other times it may be disease related such as the onset of Adult Diabetes.

Estrogen

Estrogen is not really a single hormone but a class of hormones that control things such as growth, the function of the female sex organs, secondary sexual characteristics, Calcium absorption etc. Estrogen includes hormones such as estradiol and estrone which are essential for the health of the reproductive organs, and estriol which is the predominant estrogen hormone during pregnancy. Estradiol is the main estrogen. Prior to menopause it is the dominant form of estrogen in the body. Estrone is an inactive or weak form of estrogen which the body produces after menopause in the fat tissues.

As a fetus your body began producing estrogen when you were 15 to 20 weeks old, at puberty your levels of estrogen increased dramatically and maybe even erratically and from then on your life became influenced by the cyclic monthly changes. Then along comes menopause which is kind of the reverse of adolescence.

Progesterone

Progesterone is produced mainly by the ovaries, with a small amount produced by the adrenal glands. During pregnancy the placenta produces large amounts. Progesterone is also needed for the production of other hormones such as cortisol which plays an important role in the metabolism of carbohydrates, fats and proteins and in the body's response to injury and infection. The production of ovarian progesterone declines during the menopausal years.

Follicle Stimulating Hormone (FSH) - Produced by the pituitary gland to stimulate the ovaries to get follicles growing. This is the hormone that starts the menstrual cycle.

Luteinising Hormone (LH) - Produced by the pituitary gland to get the follicle to release the egg.

Testosterone

As well as being the main hormone for men testosterone is also important to women. Half of a women's testosterone is produced in the ovaries and the other half in the adrenal glands. Testosterone helps to determine secondary sexual chrematistics such as muscle mass, patterns of hair growth and sexual desire. Testosterone levels reduce about one third in the average post-menopausal women, if the ovaries are removed the fall is twice as great.

Conclusion

With so many hormones in the body each doing their own thing but at the same time influencing many other hormones, sometimes the best way to go is to try to balance the lot of them instead of picking on individuals. This can be a great benefit especially to people prone to other problems such as Adult Onset Diabetes. The best herb to do this is Maca. This herb is known as an Adaptogen, which means it tries to adapt the body to get the best you can out of it under the present conditions. I prefer using this herb in powder form and I think it also works out cheaper this way.

Maca

Actions - Nutritive, increases energy and stamina, adaptogen, helps to restore the endocrine system eg ovaries, pancreas, thyroid, adrenals etc.

Maca is a root vegetable only grown in Peru, indigenous to the Andean Mountains. It is a turnip like tuber that has a pleasant malty butterscotch like flavor and has been used for well over 5000 years. Like other herbs grown at high altitudes in extreme weather conditions (eg - Ginseng) this herbs packs quiet a punch especially nutrition wise.

Maca strengthens and balances the endocrine system and has a positive effect on the organs which become more balanced and stronger. Areas Maca may help in are PMS, Menopause, Hot Flushes, Frigidity, Chronic Fatigue, Anemia, Infertility, Breast Feeding and much more. Some people even use it as a HRT replacement.

When shopping for Maca remember that it only comes from the Peruvian highlands and only the root of the plant is used

This little write up is only an introduction to you of Maca and how it may benefit you, I will leave it to you to do your own research. I have been using Maca on patients for years now and only really started using it for its nutrition and energy giving properties and always kind of used it as a background remedy. Now I really pay attention to it as an endocrine balancer especially to the adrenal glands. Now it's your turn to see what it can do. Being a Adaptogen this is a long term use herb give it at least 6 months so it can supply the nutrition and fine tune the body. Adaptogens adapt your body to suit you and your circumstances and this cannot be done overnight. A good rule is to use them for 3 months as this is the blood cycle, in other words the blood replaces itself every 3 months and as your hormones rely on feedback to receptors via the blood stream then this is the best time for you to stand back and judge the results.

Other Adaptogens in the Herbal - Withania, Ginseng, Siberian Ginseng and Schizandra.

Warning - Maca is very rich in nutrients so start with small doses like a quarter of a teaspoon and slowly over a few weeks build up to the recommended dose.

Notes

Gathering Information, Know Your Enemy

The most accurate way to determine if you have PMS is to keep a Menstrual Calendar on which you chart the timing of your symptoms and menstrual bleeding. It is not the type of symptoms that is important but rather the fact that your symptoms recur every month the same time after ovulation and are relieved when the menstrual bleeding is well under way. After about 3 months of using your chart if you have PMS you may notice that there is a pattern beginning to emerge and it is the same month after month, sometimes getting worse. Another advantage of using the chart is that you can tell if you are getting better from the treatment or not. This gives you control and confidence in what you are trying to achieve.

The way PMS is diagnosed is from a Menstrual Calendar so if worst came to worst and the Natural Remedies offered you no relief then you would at least have a calendar that you could give to your Doctor and as it is their main diagnostic tool for this condition they would have to begin treatment right away. It is up to you to choose which symptoms to record but the process of daily recording is essential when symptoms are noticed. Don't confuse the issue by writing down to many symptoms limit it to your 3 or 4 worst problems and use a single letter to indicate each of the 4 symptoms. Some people just put an x on the days they feel awful and a big X when it becomes unbearable. What really matters is that the chart shows up the days of your periods and the days of your problems so that it can be used for diagnosis.

It is quite normal for some women to have menstruation every 21 days and others every 36 days. There may well be variations of 3 to 4 days between the lengths of your cycles and yet these would be considered perfectly normal. Keep the chart up regularly as you try out different treatments so that you have a visual record of success or failure. Despite individual variations the cyclical nature of PMS stands out very clearly on a chart. The best way to see it is to stand back from the chart and don't focus on the letters but look at the pattern. Usually because there is not the same number of days in each month and most women usually don't have a precise 28 day cycle and the symptoms don't usually start on the same day instead of the symptoms lining up horizontally across the page they are usually diagonal.

We will use a code in plotting our chart and it will go like this.

B = Breast pain or tenderness

M = Menstrual bleeding

P = Period pain

D = Depression

H = Headache

B = Bloated, water retention

I = Irritability

F = Fatigue

For Severity - Use capitals for severe symptoms and small letters for less intense symptoms.

Feel free to add to this code any other symptom that affects you.

Download your own Chart from The Internet

Have a look on the internet as there are lots of different types of Menstrual Charts and download the one that suits you, while you are there take a look at other examples of PMS charts and see the patterns yourself. Remember every one of us is an individual and no conditions are the same but are unique to that individuals circumstances. Better still make your own, list below the main symptoms you want to cover.

Notes

Menstrual Diary Chart

Day	January	February	March	April
1	B	HBD	M	
2	B	MP	M	
3	BHBD	MP	M	
4	HBD	M		
5	HBD	M		
6	MP	M		
7	MP			
8	M			
9	M			
10	M			
11				
12				D
13				BD
14				BD
15				BD
16				BD
18				HBD
19			D	MP
20			BD	M
21			BDHBD	M
22		D	HBD	M
23		BD	MP	M
24		HBD	MP	
25		HBD	M	
26	B	HBD	M	
27	B	MP	M	
28	BD	M		
29	HBD			
30	HBD			

What If It's Not PMS

If after 2 or 3 months of charting your symptoms you find your personal chart does not match that of one with PMS don't be to disheartened for at least you are now well into your investigation and some of the changes you have made may soon start to take effect especially if you have changed your diet. There are some menstrual problems which when carefully recorded turn out not to be PMS. In fact most Medical PMS Clinics in Britain and the US will tell you that about half of all women that attend do not have PMS but suffer from some other menstrual problem. Among the common ailments masquerading as PMS are Menstrual Distress, Dysmenorrhea, Endometriosis, Postnatal Depression and Menopause. Let's now take a look at some of these and on the internet try to see what their menstrual charts look like.

Menstrual Distress

This is when symptoms are present throughout the cycle and get worse the days before the period or at the time of the period. Menstrual Distress or Menstrual Magnification as the Americans like to call it is the commonest problem found in PMS Clinics in women who don't have PMS.

The usual Consensus is that women with only mild or occasional symptoms after the period will benefit most from PMS treatment even though their problem after menstruation may remain.

Treatment

Look to the diet first and try to find your symptoms in the symptoms section and see what that has to say about it. Match the actions of herbs to your condition and see what herbs are listed under the actions, then go to the herbal and read up on those herbs and from them pick the most suitable. Read the write up at the beginning of the herbal section on how to prescribe herbs.

Dysmenorrhea

Dysmenorrhea simply means painful menstruation and there are two different types one being Spasmodic Dysmenorrhea and the other Congestive Dysmenorrhea.

Spasmodic Dysmenorrhea

These are due to uncoordinated contractions of opposing muscles in the uterus causing cramp and are most common in young women usually disappearing after childbirth. The pain usually starts just before menstrual bleeding or with it and may continue for 3 to 4 days varying from mild to excruciating pain. Other symptoms may be bowel problems, shivering or sweating, general weakness or tiredness, aching all over, back and leg pain or nausea and faintness. The pain usually eases gradually over the next 10 years and as mentioned before it usually disappears after a full term pregnancy.

Treatment

Low levels of Calcium may lead to cramping, try

taking a supplement of 500mgs daily for 10 days before a period. At time of cramping you could take Mag Phos in the Cell Salts dissolved in a wine glass of warm to hot water. Look at diet and at PMS (P). Athletes now use Magnesium Rehydration Formulas for cramps especially of bike races. You can buy these in one dose sachets and they work well in cases of cramping pains. Chamomile tea give high doses of Magnesium and Calcium in liquid form that is assimilated fast and easily in the body.

Herbal Treatment

Antispasmodic and analgesic herbs can provide relief of the symptoms but longer term treatment would include uterine toners and hormone balancers.

An example formula might be Squaw Vine, Black and Blue Cohosh and Chamomile or even Wild Yam and we can't forget Cramp Bark.

Congestive Dysmenorrhea

Pain starts well before the period and is often due to inflammatory problems with the uterus such as endometriosis, fibroids, pelvic inflammatory disease or problems with the ovary such as ovarian cysts. Pain is due to congestion in the pelvic area. It usually occurs latter in reproductive life after the age of 30 or after childbirth. The major symptoms are feelings of aching heaviness in the lower abdomen and legs, the thighs may be especially painful. Accompanying diarrhea is not uncommon. The discomfort is usually relieved once bleeding starts.

Treatment

This really depends on the cause but diet is always the best way to start. See PMS (P). If confused see a specialist to try and find a cause as it may be an infection.

Herbal Treatment

Herbal alteratives and cleaners are used here along with decongestants and Hormonal Balancers if there is PMS. An herbal formula could be Black Cohosh, Dong Quai, Ginger Dandelion and we would add Vitex as a hormone balancer if there were PMS symptoms.

Endometriosis

This pathological condition causes pain before and throughout menstruation and is accompanied by painful intercourse, pain on moving the uterus when under examination and infertility. The cells which form the lining of the womb are normally shed through the vagina during each menstruation are called endometrial cells. Sometimes these cells find their way outside the womb in places such as the outside wall of the womb or anywhere close by such as the bladder, fallopian tubes or rectum. When menstruation occurs these cells cannot be shed like normal cells through the vagina but instead form cysts which can gradually expand with each menstruation causing increased pain This happens because the wrongly placed cells still receive the messenger hormones telling them that menstruation has begun but being in the wrong place they have no way out. One of the main symptoms is severe pain during the period that cannot be relieved by over the counter analgesics. The pain often spreads to the back and down the thighs and may get worse towards the end of the period. If the bowel is involved passing motions may be painful. This condition is usually diagnosed through laparoscopy when a small viewing instrument is inserted through the abdomen. Orthodox treatment is removal by surgery or laser but the condition tends to reoccur.

Treatment

As you can see this is a hard one to treat and an Herbalist would have to sit down and think really hard about this one but the treatment would be based on the personal symptoms of the patient.

Menopause

The menopause is a natural physiological state marking the shutdown of the reproductive system and the end of child bearing. The usual age for menopause is between 45 and 55 years. Menopause can have the symptoms of hot flushes and night sweats, dryness of the vagina that causes painful sex, thinning of the layer of fat under the skin so that wrinkles and crow's feet appear and maybe some symptoms of depression. Women who have not had many problems with menstruation during their lives tend to have no problems at menopause while the ones that have had lots of problems tend to have problems during menopause.

PMS Symptoms

Because there are such a variety of symptoms in PMS the symptoms were categorized and put into 4 groupings which not only matched the symptoms but had some relevance to different levels of certain hormones as well. The biggest drawback as every woman with PMS would recognize is that the symptoms rarely fall into such tidy categories. These categories are getting less and less important now as the modern Psychiatric Drugs are getting better especially the serotonin adjusting ones but for someone like me who is trying to treat holistically using gentle methods like Homoeopathy to adjust the levels of certain hormone groupings symptoms are important. Latter on when we get into treatment with herbs you will see how important they are there to.

I feel using these groupings is probably the fastest and easiest way to teach and that it will also be helpful to you especially when deciding how to manage these symptoms.

Symptom Grading

There are four common types of PMS known as A,B,C, and D or Anxiety , Bloating , Cravings and Depression. We are now going to go into detail about each one of these so you can decide which one relates the closest to you. I have added a 5th grouping which I will call PMS (P) with the P for Pain.

PMS (A) - Anxiety
Main Symptoms
Anxiety

Irritability

Mood swings

PMS (A): Other symptoms commonly mentioned **are** anger, crying for no reason, verbally and sometimes physically abusive, feeling out of control and nervous tension. Sometimes here the symptoms can become progressively worse as the period nears. 65 to 75% of women suffer from this type mainly with the main symptoms mentioned.

PMS (B) - Bloating
Main Symptoms
Fluid retention

Weight gain

Breast tenderness

Abdominal tenderness

Swollen hands and feet

PMS (B): With the main symptoms of fluid retention effects 65 to 72% of women, there may be weight gain , abdominal bloating, breast swelling and tenderness, swollen ankles and facial swelling and with some headaches.

PMS (C) - Cravings
Main Symptoms
Food cravings

Headache
Fatigue
Dizziness
Palpitations

PMS (C): Effects 25 to 35% of women. The effects of this type are similar to hypoglycemia. The exact mechanism is not known but it seems that the blood sugar levels swing between high and low. High intake levels of coffee, tea, chocolate and alcohol in an attempt to help the situation seem only to escalate the problem especially if the diet is high in refined carbohydrates and sugar. In the absence of caffeine and other stimulants the body produces excess adrenaline which also causes anxiety, palpitations, sweating and shakiness.

PMS (D) - Depression
Main Symptoms
Depression
Crying
Forgetfulness
Confusion
Insomnia

PMS (D): Effects 25 to 37% of women. Often associated with PMS (A) which it usually follows causing symptoms of depression, weepiness, confusion, clumsiness and lack of concentration?

PMS (P) - Pain
Main Symptoms
Aches and Pains
Period Pain
Reduced Pain Threshold

PMS (P): In this category of PMS the major problem is an increased sensitivity to pain which is believed to be caused by prostaglandin imbalance. Causes are thought to be elevated estrogen levels or eating too much animal fats.

Symptoms In Detail

Here we are going to look into the symptoms and probable causes in detail and offer a range of treatments that will hopefully bring relief. Treatments looked at will be nutrition in the form of supplements and diet which we will go into more later on. Treatment with Herbs will be dealt with later but for ease of reference a lot of herbs are listed here so you can quickly check them out in the herbal at the back. Our last form of Treatment is Homoeopathy using the 4 Homoeopathic Complexes, 2 of these Complexes have Hormones in them that have been Homeopathically prepared in 2 separate potencies one low and the other higher and they are used in an attempt to adjust the levels of the hormones they are targeted to by tricking them to think that the hormone that is to low, needs raising and the hormone that is high needs lowering. Other Homoeopathic remedies in the Complexes help counter the symptoms common to the type of PMS suffered.

Notes

PMS (A) - Anxiety

Main Symptoms

Anxiety, Irritability, Mood swings, Nervous Tension

Causes

High estrogen, leads to excess adrenaline and serotonin. Low progesterone.

PMS (A) : 65 to 75% of women suffer from this type. Excess estrogen in relation to progesterone and sometimes even a deficiency in progesterone causes an imbalance in brain chemicals (serotonin, adrenaline and dopamine) which over stimulates and brings on the symptoms of anxiety, nervous tension etc. and mental relaxation is inhibited.

This condition also blocks the metabolism of vitamin B6 and leads to poor metabolism of the essential fatty acids in the body. In this case the minerals magnesium, chromium and zinc will be depleted and there is an increased need for vitamins C and B as well as B6. Because of this blood sugar levels are affected especially when the diet is poor and may lead to symptoms of HYPOGLYCAEMIA (See PMS (C)) with possible associated mood changes. Magnesium and zinc supplements may help as well as a balanced natural food diet.

Nutritional Treatment

A diet high in fat and low in fiber can increase the levels of estrogen in the system and another point to think about is that in one major survey Caffeine consumption was 2 and a half times higher in PMS suffers compared to non-sufferers. Let's take a look at some of the symptoms of excess Caffeine they are Anxiety, irritability, headaches, increased urination, and insomnia and in some palpations oh e heart. Another point to ponder on is that high levels of estrogen slow down the rate that caffeine is broken down by the liver. Cutting out caffeine is one of the first things to try, remember on average a mug of tea contains 100 to 130mgs of caffeine and coffee between 150 to 250 mgs of caffeine.

Supplements

B Complex - To support the nerves, brain chemistry and adrenal glands. B vitamins are involved with the livers handling of estrogen and the production of dopamine a brain chemical.

B6 - Take the B Complex but let's say an hour latter take B6 on its own for a few months and see what happens. B6 can aid in restoring estrogen levels to normal and acts as a coenzyme in many hormonal reactions. B6 is essential for the manufacture of the brain chemicals serotonin and dopamine and the pill may increase the bodies need.

Vitamin C - Helps rid the body of excess estrogen.

Vitamin E - Helps relieve nervous tension and irritability.

Magnesium - A lack of this can lead to nervous tension and heart palpitations.

L Tyrosine - Reduces anxiety, headaches and depression.

Tryptophan (Amino Acid) - May significantly reduce irritability, tension and mood swings.

Zinc - An important mineral for the reproductive system.

See Supplement Section In General

Herbal Treatment

Progestogenic Herbs - Chaste berry, Sarsaparilla, Wild Yam.

Estrogenic Herbs - Red clover, Sage, Licorice, Black Cohosh, Motherwort if coming to menopause.

Nervines or Sedatives - Skullcap, Valerian, Passion Flower, Vervain, Chamomile.

Others - Withania for anxiety and exhaustion. False and True Unicorn Root and Squaw Vine.

Suggested formula for A with fluid retention.

Skullcap

Chaste Berry

Dandelion leaf

False Unicorn Root

Look up the individual Herbs in the Herbal Section

Homoeopathic Complex PMS(A)

Based on the symptoms of anxiety, irritability, mood swings and nervous tension.

Estrogen (minis), Progesterone (plus), Chamomile , Sepia , Nux Vom , Kali Mur 6X

PMS (B) - Bloating

Main Symptoms - Breast tenderness, Abdominal Bloating, Swollen hands and feet.

Causes - Fluid retention, High Aldosterone, Weight gain, High estrogen.

PMS (B): This type which the main symptom is fluid retention effects 65 to 72% of women, there may be weight gain, abdominal bloating , breast swelling and tenderness, swollen ankles and facial swelling. High estrogen levels disrupt the normal output of aldosterone which regulates fluid balance causing salt and water retention. It is worsened by a high excretion of magnesium by the kidneys. Daily supplements that may help include magnesium, Vit E, Primrose Oil, Vit B6 and those Mentioned in PMS (A). Salt in the diet should be strictly avoided at this time.

Nutritional Treatment

Symptoms due to excess fluid can easily be made worse by a poor diet. A high intake of sodium is the commonest cause of fluid retention in women. Try to reduce salt intake and be especially aware of processed foods as they are usually loaded with salt, another idea is to change to Vegetable Salt instead of the normal Table Salt. Plain fruit and vegetables, meat, fish, beans and rice are all low in sodium and have good levels of potassium. Potassium counters sodium in the body and works like this, cells use potassium to draw fluid to them while the blood uses sodium to draw fluid to it so between them both a balance is maintained. A good natural diet used for reducing weight has been found to relieve the symptoms of fluid retention.

Supplements (see PMS(A))

B6 - Reduces water retention and aids in restoring estrogen to normal levels.

Vitamin C - Helps to rid the body of excess estrogen and also aids in the relief of breast swelling.

Vitamin E - Can help reduce breast tenderness.

Magnesium - Deficiency can increase the levels of Aldosterone in the body.

Tryptophan - May relieve fluid retention and breast tenderness.

Primrose Oil - See supplement section.

See Supplement Section In General

Herbal Treatment

Herbal Diuretics - Dandelion leaf is one of the safest diuretics as it puts more potassium in the body then it takes out. Parsley is another good simple diuretic.

Progestogenic Herbs - Chaste Berry and Wild Yam.

Homoeopathic Complex PMS(B) Mixer

Based on symptoms of fluid retention, weight gain, breast tenderness, abdominal tenderness and swollen hands and feet.

Nat Mur 6X, Apis , Strophanthus , Apocynum.

PMS (C) - Cravings

Main Symptoms - Food cravings, Headache, Fatigue, Dizziness, Palpitations.

Causes - Similar to hypoglycemia

PMS (C) : Effects 25 to 35% of women. The effects of this type are similar to hypoglycemia. The exact mechanism is not known but it seems that the blood sugar levels swing between high and low. High intake levels of coffee, tea, chocolate and alcohol in an attempt to help the situation seem only to escalate the problem especially if the diet is high in refined carbohydrates and sugar. In the absence of caffeine and other stimulants the body produces excess adrenaline which also causes anxiety, palpitations, sweating and shakiness.

Nutritional Treatment

This often comes with PMS (A) and symptoms may be one or two weeks before the period appetite increases and cravings begin, particularly for sweet foods and chocolate with stress often making the condition worse. Some of these symptoms may be due to a fall in blood sugar called hypoglycemia. As the brain and nervous system relies on glucose for its source of energy a fall can result in a whole host of nervous system symptoms. The body compensates by producing more adrenalin which increases the levels of glucose in the blood but can aggravate the symptoms of anxiety, palpations, sweating and shaking.

Often the cravings for sweet foods, sugary snacks and chocolate are the result of an irregular and inadequate diet. What is not widely appreciated is that calorie requirements in the premenstrual week increase by up to 500 calories per day so this may be the main cause of the sweet tooth.

Women with PMS (C) may also experience headaches, fatigue, pounding heart, dizziness and fainting. These symptoms can be due to the swings in blood sugar levels and over reliance in the social stimulants - coffee, tea, chocolate, cola and cigarettes. Three good regular meals with two wholesome in between snacks and cutting down on sugar and stimulants are all essential to treat PMS (C). Blood sugar levels are also controlled by hormones with the main 2 being Insulin which lowers the blood sugar levels and Glucagon which raises the blood sugar levels. As you may be beginning to see hormones don't work in isolation and they all affect each other. When Insulin levels are constantly kept to high by a diet rich in sugar and refined carbohydrates this causes high levels of free circulating estrogens which because they are not bound do damage to estrogen sensitive tissues such as the breast tissue which could lead to cancers..

If you have a problem stabilizing your blood sugar you may want to supplement chromium or try the herb Fenugreek.

Supplements
B Complex.

Chromium - Helps to improve efficient use of insulin and keep blood sugar levels steady. Take 100 to 200 micrograms once or twice a day.

Magnesium - This mineral is often deficient in women who consume a diet that is high in refined carbohydrates and sugar

Glutamine (Amino Acid) - Helps to improve mental clarity, fatigue, reduces blood sugar, reduces sugar cravings, alleviates aggressiveness, improves mood, improves concentration and lifts depression. Take 500 to 1000mg twice daily for 3 months.

Tryptophan (Amino Acid) - May give relief to headaches.

Primrose Oil - See supplement section.

See Supplement Section In General

Herbal Treatment

Licorice - To balance blood sugar levels and support adrenal glands.

Fenugreek - Coats the intestines so there is a mechanical barrier which slows down the release of sugars into the blood.

Gymnemia – Helps stabilize the blood sugar and may help with sugar cravings especially if the tincture touches the tongue.

Fringe Tree for the pancreas.

Homoeopathic Complex PMS(C) Mixer

For the symptoms of food cravings, headache, fatigue, dizziness, palpitations.

Nat Mur 6X, sepia , Conium , Cyclamen.

PMS (D) - Depression

Main Symptoms – Depression, Crying, Forgetfulness, Confusion, Insomnia

Causes - Low estrogen, High progesterone, High aldosterone (controls fluid balance)

PMS (D) : Effects 25 to 37% of women. This type appears to be due to a high level of progesterone in relation to estrogen with the progesterone acting as depressant causing symptoms of depression, weepiness, confusion, clumsiness and lack of concentration. Low levels of estrogen are thought to aggravate the symptoms by breaking down mood enhancing chemicals. (Excess lead in the blood makes this worse). Vitamins B1 and B6 help counteract the symptoms.

Nutritional Treatment

Depression can be a common premenstrual symptom and usually comes along with other premenstrual symptoms. Some studies have found that those most likely to suffer from it are more often overweight and do less exercise then those who do not suffer with this problem. It is also known that in people with severe depression the chance of finding some degree of B Vitamin deficiency is much higher than would be expected in the general population.

This form of PMS may be caused by a to low level of estrogen in the blood and sometimes a diet high in fiber can remove the building blocks of hormones thus reducing the amount of hormones in the system.

Declining levels of estrogen as you head closer to menopause also seem to be correlated with a higher vulnerability to depression and anxiety disorders.

If you suffer from depression scrutinize your diet to make sure your blood sugar levels remain as constant as possible. If you have a problem stabilizing your blood sugar you may want to supplement chromium or try the herb Fenugreek.

Supplements

Chromium - Helps to improve efficient use of insulin and keeps blood sugar levels steady Take 100 to 200 micrograms once or twice a day..

Tryptophan 500mg (Amino Acid) - Can help with some types of depression. See supplement section.

Glutamine (Amino Acid) - Helps to improve mental clarity, fatigue, reduces blood sugar, reduces sugar cravings, alleviates aggressiveness, improves mood, improves concentration and lifts depression. Take 500 to 1000mg twice daily for 3 months.

B6, B12 and B Complex - See supplement section.
See Supplement Section In General

Herbal Treatment

Estrogenic Herbs - Red clover, Sage, Licorice, Black Cohosh, Motherwort if coming to menopause.
Antidepressive Herbs - Damiana, Rosemary, Skullcap ,St Johns Wort, Valerian, Vervain.
Other Herbs – Blue Cohosh, Withania, Panax Ginseng, and liver herbs such as Milk Thistle and

Dandelion.

Homoeopathic Complex PMS(D)

For the symptoms of depression, crying, forgetfulness, confusion and insomnia.

Estrogen (plus), Progesterone (minis), Puls , Ignatia , Nat Mur 6X, Sepia.

PMS (P) - Pain

Main Symptoms - Aches and Pains, Period Pain, Reduced Pain Threshold

Causes – May be a diet high in animal fat. May be high estrogen Levels

In this category of PMS the major problem is an increased sensitivity to pain which is believed to be caused by prostaglandin imbalance. Causes are thought to be elevated estrogen levels or eating too much animal fat.

Nutritional Treatment

Essential fatty acids are the building blocks for Prostaglandins which are powerful hormone like chemicals that regulate many vital body functions such as hormone production, circulation, immune function and inflammation among many others. There are 3 Different Families of Prostaglandins which we will lay out in chart form for you.

Prostaglandin Family

Prostaglandin 1 - Gamma Linolenic Acid (GLA). One of the good ones. Reduces pain and inflammation

Food Sources - Sesame, Sunflower seeds and oil, cold pressed vegetable oils, Black currant seeds and oil, Borage Oil, Evening Primrose Oil.

Prostaglandin 2 - Arachidonic Acid. One of the bad ones. Increases pain and inflammation, can result in sticky blood platelets and poor circulation

Food Sources - Saturated animal fats in meats especially in red meat, full cream dairy products, preserved meats, fried food, processed and takeaway meals.

Prostaglandin 3 - Alpha linolenic Acid and Eicosapentaenoic Acid. One of the good ones. Reduces pain and inflammation

Food sources - Linseed oil, Black Currant seeds and oil, Fish Oils like Cod, Mackerel, tuna, salmon, sardines.

PMS pains can be reduced and may even be relieved by removing or cutting down on the bad fats (Listed in Prostaglandin 2) and increasing consumption of the good ones and even supplementing some of the good ones with the more popular being Evening Primrose Oil and the Fish Oils.

Supplements

Evening Primrose Oil, Fish Oils and other oils and foods listed in the table above.

Magnesium - Reduces sensitivity to pain in doses of 200 to 800mgs daily.

Herbal Treatment

Anti-inflammatory Herbs - Black Cohosh, Blue Cohosh, Chamomile, Feverfew, Ginger, Lady's Mantle, St Johns Wort, Sage, Wild Yam, Withania.

Analgesic Herbs - Chamomile, Dong Quai, Hops, Lady's Mantle, Passion Flower, St Johns Wort, Skullcap, Valerian, Wild Yam, Withania.

Feverfew is a prostaglandin inhibitor and may help with period pain and migraine headache if taken for a long term.

Notes

Premenstrual Dysphoric Disorder (PMDD)

The term PMDD is another way of saying really severe PMS. Dysphoric means a sense of disquiet, restlessness, or malaise. The condition used to be called Late Luteal Phase Disorder but has now been changed. For about 3 - 8% of the women, the cyclical symptoms are so severe that they interfere with their daily functioning and personal relationships.as the mood changes are major shifts, and are extremely difficult to live with. The symptoms are usually strongly emotional, characterized by mood swings, depression, and anxiety along with physical symptoms. Many women feel overwhelmed or out of control. With some fearing they may hurt themselves and their loved ones.

PPMD can arise at any age but often appears in the mid-20s and gets worse before menopause. The symptoms disappear during pregnancy and after menopause which point to this being a problem caused by the menstrual cycle. This condition is not fully understood but it is believed that it is a brain chemistry problem which results in mood and behavioral distress. They think the fluctuating levels of estrogen and progesterone may affect the brains serotonin levels with a decreased supply during the luteal phase.

The most effective treatments for this condition seem to enhance serotonin activity. We will have to wait for more research to be done before we get any better answers. Again as in PMS your best and only diagnostic tool is the Menstrual Diary Chart. I have an idea though, I will try to explain, I doubt if it will be a cure but I believe it will help. I mentioned before the herb Maca which is in a class of herbs known as Adaptogens. In other words they may not cure but try to adapt you to your condition so you can get the best out of yourself. I use these a lot in people with cancer especially those undergoing chemo therapy (Astragalus). Maca as mentioned before is an endocrine balancer. The endocrine system is basically any gland that squirts a hormone eg ovaries, thyroid, adrenal glands etc. Just reading these few lines gives you the reason why I suggested Maca for PMS. In being a Medical Herbalist we are trained to think in actions. Adaptogen is an herbal action; its action is as previously mentioned. When we want to make a chosen action stronger we add to our formula herbs strong in that action. A good example is putting 3 or 4 strong anti-inflammatory herbs together in a formula for the treatment of Rheumatism. The Adaptogen herb that I am thinking of for PPMD is Withania as it has an action on the brain chemistry and I use this herb a lot in PMS.(P) or in any condition of pain especially in the chronic pains of cancer or any condition of severe chronic pain. To sum up think of Maca for endocrine balancing and nutrition. Withania is stress, pain, brain chemistry, breast cancer (antitumor) and miscarriages.

The Liver And PMS

The liver plays a very important part in the body as it screens all the blood and takes out the rubbish and also acts as a big chemical warehouse by storing lots of chemicals and nutrients that may be needed for some job in the future. The liver specializes in breaking down and deactivating toxins which is one of its main jobs. Our modern lifestyles gives the liver a very hard time as most of the foods we eat are not natural but mostly processed and filled with chemicals, then we might go out and have a few drinks which loads up the liver more because now it's got to pull down all these alcohol molecules as well as sort out dinner. When you really start feeling the effects of the alcohol you know the liver is having a hard time catching up with you, and then what about all the exhaust fumes you breathe in on the way home the livers got to deal with that to. So now you can see the liver is one of the hardest working and most abused organs in the body. Well by now you're wondering what this has to do with PMS well the answer is that all the hormones in your blood circulation get pulled down and deactivated by the liver.

If the liver slows down and gets behind this can throw a spanner in the works because some hormones that should of been deactivated hasn't been and is causing something to work that shouldn't be and etc etc it's like a domino effect. I have actually seen a good example of this in a man who was dying of slow liver failure , because the liver was failing it wasn't breaking down estrogen (men make this to but in small amounts) and he was slowly developing breasts and getting other feminine features.

If you think you are giving your liver a hard time then stop as sometimes this alone can stop or ease the symptoms of PMS. Try a liver cleansing diet or just eat natural foods, stop smoking and cut back on the drinking and try to get some stress out of your life as this helps too.

Eat foods which help the liver correctly process estrogens especially those that contain methionine (a sulphurous amino acid) which is found in beans, eggs, onions and garlic. To help your liver function eat some of these foods when you can - endive, chicory, silver beat, outer leaves of cos lettuce, dandelion leaf, dandelion root, grapefruit and any other bitter tasting foods as the bitter tasting foods prime the whole digestive process and stimulate the increased flow of bile which is the vehicle for removing the substances broken down by the liver cells in other words the waste of the liver.

In Traditional Chinese Medicine symptoms of liver disharmony include irritability, depression, frustration, anger, digestive upsets and common gynecological complaints such as PMS, irregular periods, no periods, infertility and period pain.

To Protect Liver Cells

1/.Milk Thistle - Contains the most potent liver cell

protective compounds known to exist.

2/.Antioxidants - Such as vitamins A,E and C, beta carotene and selenium.

3/.Lecithin - A major component of cell membranes. Protects liver cell membranes from damage from the continual attack of toxins and free radicals.

Herbal Actions And Herbs Affecting The Liver

Hepatics - Are Herbs that tone and strengthen the liver, and may increase the flow of bile which is the waste product of the liver and a natural laxative.

Herbs - Agrimony, <u>Dandelion</u>, Motherwort, Milk Thistle, Shizandra, Vervain, Yarrow.

Cholagogues - Stimulate the release of bile from the gallbladder which can relieve gallbladder problems, bile is also the body's natural laxative so cholagogues have a laxative effect as well.

Herbs - Dandelion, Milk Thistle.

How To Rid The Body Of Too Much Estrogen

As mentioned above it is the livers job to pull down the excess hormones and to rid them from the body. We shall continue here from where we left off. Bile is the livers waste product and carries in it most of the building blocks of what the liver has just pulled down and other waste products. Bile leaves the liver and is stored in the gallbladder were it awaits its second function which is in the digestive process. Bile is secreted into the intestines through a pipe line at the beginning of the small intestines and functions as a detergent to fats spreading them out into ever smaller drops to allow for easier absorption, another function of bile is that it is the body's natural laxative and the brown color of fasces is from the bile it contains. Pale whitish colored stools are a sign of a blocked bile duct.

Now we come to the Catch 22 of the digestive system and it is this. The small intestines work on a united we stand and dived we fall policy which works like this. Food goes into the small intestines and is spread along its length by water which divides and separates the particles for easier absorption. The food leaves the small intestines with most of the absorption taken place and enters the large intestine whose main function is to reabsorb the water and recycle it.

The problem is that not only has the food been absorbed but to a certain degree so has the bile that entered form the gallbladder and all those bits and pieces of pulled down hormones have now re-entered the system. So how do we prevent this from happening? We will answer that soon buts lets now look at the symptoms of too much Estrogen in the system.

Symptoms Of To High Estrogen

Heavier than usual periods, longer than usual periods, PMS. Estrogen excess is also linked to endometriosis, fibroids, fibrocystic breast disease, breast and endometrial cancer.

What Can We Do.

The answer is to increase the FIBER in our diets. The bulk of fiber travelling through the system binds bile to it and escorts it out of the body. Bowel health is intimately linked to hormone health and fiber intake is essential to ensure healthy bowel movements. Women on high fiber diets such as vegetarians have considerably lower levels of estrogens circulating in their blood. Fiber also helps to regulate blood sugar levels which can help with premenstrual cravings. There is now clear evidence that high fiber diets significantly reduce other hormonal problems such as premenstrual problems and may in time save you from hormone related cancers such as breast cancer. We eat on average 9 to 10 grams of fiber daily and the authorities recommend we double this while other experts such as the National Cancer Institute in the US recommend even higher levels of 25 to 35 grams per day. Simply put if you include at least 4 pieces of fruit, a bowel of muesli or porridge, a couple of slices of wholemeal bread and a generous portion of beans, peas or lintels in your diet daily you should reach the 25 to 35 grams level.

Fiber Rich Foods

1/.Legumes - Beans, peas, pulses, lentils and chick peas are rich sources of fiber.
2/.Wholegrains are fiber rich - Porridge, muesli, wholemeal breads, buckwheat, brown rice etc.
3/.Fruits and Vegetables 5 to 7 portions a day - Pears,

raspberries, figs, prunes, bananas, dried apricots, dates, plums, olives, sweet potatoes, mangoes, yams, cabbage, nuts and seeds.

4/. Added Fiber - Oat fiber, rice fiber, psyllum husks, freshly ground linseeds. Build up fiber content slowly especially if you have digestive problems as the body does not like fast changes.

Notes

Introduction To Iridology

I have now been using Iridology for over 20 years and it has been a great help to me and to the many thousands I have helped with it in that time. I have a great love of Iridology as it is like being a Detective gathering all the clues and putting it all together and arriving to your conclusions. After doing it for so long your intuition gets well developed and can lead you to insights that you would never have expected. It also ruins your love life as you look into their eyes and think my god they've got this and that. I will now tell you of the two most memorable occasions I had with Iridology both of these happened over a decade ago. One was in a big open market on a Sunday where I used to do Iridology. A lady about 50 asked me to look at her eyes and tell her what I could see for she had recently had a few problems. So putting on my Detectives cap I got to work and got so confused I had to give up. I could see massive trauma to the lungs, then the same to the digestive system, the poor liver had taken a beating along with the kidneys. I was at a loss as to what could do so much damage to so many systems in such a short time. I told her what I had seen and why I was so confused, I said you're lucky to be alive. She looked at me and laughed and said that's what my Doctor said. First she had the lung problem and ended up in hospital, then the digestive problems and went back again. Next was the Kidney problems and back to hospital again. The last time in hospital the Doctor said I think someone's trying to kill you. To cut a long story short a Private Detective was put on the case finding her husband had insured her for a few million dollars without her knowing. She's now divorced happy and healthy. Another time was when I was giving a Lecture at a Buddhist Conference Center, after the lecture it was arranged for me to do the eyes of a whole lot of people. On one lady I found a diamond shape right on the heart, this is a sign that you really don't want to find. You can't really say your hearts had it or is broken as that is a bit like the witch doctor pointing the bone so you have to be very careful. I am used to this now because you can't tell all you see and think especially when there is nothing the patient can really do about it, so I kind of go round in circles and slowly get the information I need. I found that a short while ago she was having very bad heart palpitations and pains in the heart. She had got scared and gone to the Doctor but they could find nothing wrong. No one in her family had heart problems and she was only in her early 30s and seemed fit and well and the rest of her eyes told me she was a healthy and very strong person. There were no obvious symptoms of heart failure. So confused I asked when did all this start happening and what do you think was the cause. Then she started crying. She had a large young family and her husband whom she loved had run off with another lady and said he was never coming back. She had been betrayed, she really did have a broken heart. I have now seen this about 3 times now since she educated me and now pay very close attention to what stress, emotions and shock can do to the body. On the others the heartbreak had happened years ago and on all of them there were no healing signs, it looked as though the wound was there to stay.

The Beginning Of Iridology

The basics of Iridology were first put in print in 1670 by a Dresden Doctor named Philippus Meyens in his book Chiromatica Medica. These basics were later expanded by Ignatz Von Peczely (1826 - 1911) who became known as the father of Iridology.

At the age of 11 Ignatz was trying to free an owl trapped in his garden when he accidentally broke one of its legs. He soon noticed the appearance of a dark stripe in the lower part of the birds eye. Ignatz dressed the owl's leg, nursed it to health and released it when it was well. Upon recovery the owl decided to take up residence in the garden and Ignatz observed through time the appearance of white and crooked lines (Healing Lines) over the black stripe. The event made a strong impression on the boy and remained in his memory.

At the age of 20 Ignatz became involved in the Hungarian Revolt of 1846 in which he was wounded and then imprisoned until 1853. I personally believe this is where he got all his theories into shape though not much is historically documented about him and he only wrote one book. To explain it quickly when you are severely injured by a nerve reflex a mark is put in the iris of the eye. Say you have been shot in the leg, then a mark will appear in the eye at about six o'clock and it will look a bit like a bullet hole through glass. You would also see this sign from a fracture of the leg as well. I have seen these signs in many veterans and have been told by some that they have seen them in the eyes of the dead. Using this fact you can see it would be fairly easy to work out an iris chart in 7 years of jail checking out the relations between your wounds and your other wounded prisoners. Medical operations do not leave marks in the Iris for during these anesthetic is used and the nervous system is shut down and is thus unable to leave a mark in the iris. Here I always look at the area where the organ was removed to see if it was actually unhealthy before it was taken out and many times it seems alright.

The birth of Iridology is said to have been about 1861 for at this time Ignatz was having great success with Iridology and people were coming far and wide for his help. At about this time he came to the attention of the Local Authorities Doctors Quack Hit Squad who promptly paid him a visit with the Doctor in charge confronting him and calling him a Quack whereupon Ignatz looked into his eyes and replied you have suffered from such and such disease which has been falsely treated to which the Doctor admitted and did not speak further of fraud but he was made to undergo medical training.

Ignatz began training to become a Doctor at the age of 36 at the Medical College in Vienna and received his degree in 1867. While serving his internship he continued his research into Iridology by studying the patients especially ones with traumatic wounds and also performed many autopsies confirming the existence of ailments he had seen in the iris before the patient died. Doctor Von Peczely book Discoveries In The Realms Of Nature And Art Of Healing was published in 1880.

So as we can see from the above Ignatz discovered much about body positions in the iris and what certain signs mean. Now we move on to the man who discovered what different colors in the iris mean. From positions, signs and colors you have modern Iridology for the 3 combined is how you practice Iridology.

In 1859 an eight year old boy named Nils Liljequist in Stockholm Sweden began taking an interest in the irises of his own eyes. At the age of 14 he was diagnosed with malaria and treated with iodine and as the years went on he noticed the color of his eyes where changing, going from blue to green. In 1871 at the age of 20 he published a paper titled Quinine and Iodine Change The Color Of The Iris. This observation lead him to see that different drugs and elements can cause color changes in the iris. Bernard Jensen is the modern day Iridologist who started putting everything together and it is his chart that I have used for over the years and have found it to be very accurate. Get on google and download his Iridology chart or head off to your library for a book on Iridology, some of them have a reversed chart that you can use for your own eyes looking in the mirror.

Iridology And PMS

You can find a lot about PMS using Iridology. Usually the first sign I see in an eye of someone with PMS are nerve rings or their proper name Nuero Vascular Cramp Rings. These look like this. ((@)).The a is the pupil, the circle is called the nerve wreath and sits about one third out from the pupil and the area where the brackets are the colored part of the eye ending in the white. Nerve rings look like the brackets but they can be on the top and the bottom only or as well. Most Police and most Ambulance personal whose eyes I have looked into over the years have 2 to 3 nerve rings. That's just the stress of the Job. 5 to 6 nerve rings and you're probably going to have a nervous breakdown. You use nerve rings as a gauge to stress levels as they can come and go fast. I have a big magnified shaving mirror which is always in my briefcase and when I find nerve rings in someone's eyes I show them and as they are look I shine my torch sideways across the eye which kind of makes it look 3 dimensional and the rings turn into waves as you can see the up and down of them. I tell them that the rings mean stress. The more you get the more stressed you are. The less you get the less stressed you are. The balls now in your court, you've got the gauge now so you know when and if you're getting better or not. I explain to them when you are stressed you are like this and I hold up my hands and clench my fists and tighten my body, the more stressed you are the tighter you clench your fists and body, they eventually get the picture. When you are clenched up that tight the nervous system is using massive amounts of Calcium and Magnesium which is what the nerves run on and also the muscles. The more stressed you are the more you will burn. The more stressed you are the more adrenaline you will be using which will be depleting all your B vitamins. A nervous breakdown results more from the depletion of Calc, Mag and the Bs from the body then from the stress for if you supplemented them you would have gone on for a lot longer. Another mistake people make is that they don't realize that the B vitamins are water soluble so when they take a dose most of it passes out through the urine giving it that fluorescent color, so try to find a slow release B vitamin so your urine will be funny colored all day.

Next we check out the reproductive organs. Look at the chart and you will see that you have the right and left eye. The left eye does the left hand side of the body while the right does the right side of the body. First we start by looking at the ovaries. I am always weary of the dual organs such as the ovaries, kidneys, lungs and thyroid because if one is not working well the other usually tries to compensate. A good example of this is the kidneys where one side could nearly be dead and withered away while the other side has compensated and grown twice the normal size. According to the doctors there is nothing wrong with the poor person, see have a look at the blood test results, all are giving perfect readings there's nothing wrong. I could say a few more nasty things but I shall control myself. But let's focus on the poor patient for there are many who have suffered like this including myself and no doubt more than a few of my readers. So check both ovaries. Iridology only shows you tissue changes and doesn't tell you what's wrong, that's where playing the detective comes in but at least you have a clue that something is not right in that area. Another common mark I see in the eyes of women falls between the areas of the vagina where it joins the uterus so on the chart it's where the cervix is. It's the size of a pinhead and the color is a kind of orange reddish. This is usually from a strong birth control pill and is actually a drug spot. These spots usually settle where a drug is targeted at. The most important area to check for PMS is the pituitary gland for this gland controls most of the hormones in the body. I also check the thyroid area especially for those with fatigue. Iridology has greatly enriched my life and through it I have empowered others and taught them how to see if they are getting better or not thus putting their own health back into their own hands. I hope this introduction to Iridology inspires you to use it for yourself to improve your own health.

Supplements For PMS

Vitamins

1/. **Vitamin A** and Beta Carotene help to sooth and heal the mucous membranes of the body. Vitamin A can also reduce excessive bleeding and thus help prevent anemia. Deficiencies have been linked to PMS.

Food Sources - Apricots, carrots, green leafy vegetables, liver, mint, egg yolk.

2/. **Cod Liver Oil** - Good sources of vitamins A and D. You need Vitamin D and sunlight for the assimilation of calcium.

3/. **Vitamin B6 (Pyridoxine).** A number of studies have found that B6 in a daily dosage of 25 to 100mg can give satisfactory relief too many PMS symptoms such as premenstrual headaches, fluid retention, irritability, and depression in around 60 to 80% of women. B6 helps to regulate the brains biochemistry and is necessary for the conversion of tryptophan to the brain hormone serotonin. Serotonin is a natural regulator of mood, sex drive, sleep and appetite.

Food Sources - Brewer's yeast, raw nuts and seeds, pith of citrus fruits (marmalade).

4/. **B 12** can also be of benefit. It may be a good idea to buy B6 and B12 and use them by themselves for a while or at least a container full so you can observe the effect on yourself.

B12 and **Folic acid** can help to improve energy levels.

If fatigue and or depression are a problem take 250 to 500micrograms of B12 and 800micrograms of Folic Acid daily.

Food Sources - Clams, egg yolk, herring, liver, meat, milk, oysters, salmon, sardines.

5/. B Complex - If you are taking B6 or B12 or experimenting with them to see if they work for you make sure you do not take them at the same time as the B Complex, try to keep them a couple of hours apart. This complex is good for the nerves and adrenal glands.

6/. Hesperidin or Bioflavonoids - Bioflavonoids have been used successfully to reduce hot flashes as well as to reduce heavy bleeding. They also help protect and strengthen capillary walls. Take 500mgs 3 times daily with 500mgs of Vitamin C as long as you have symptoms. The main bioflavonoids are rutin, quercetin, citrin, hesperidin, genestein and diadzein.

Food Sources - Buck wheat, citrus fruit, sprouts, skins of fruits, vegetables and soy products.

7/. Vitamin E - Involved in the production of some of the pituitary and adrenal hormones. Helps to relieve breast problems, nervous tension, fatigue, depression, is a very potent anti-oxidant, lack of vitamin E can cause excessive or scanty periods, reduced sexual desire and some skin problems.

Food sources - Wheat germ oil and all cold pressed oils from vegetable sources, sesame seeds, sunflower and pumpkin seeds, hazel nuts, walnuts, peanuts, sprouted seeds, spinach, Brussel sprouts, brown rice, asparagus, celery, peas, avocado.

Caution - No one taking anticoagulant drugs for thrombosis or other similar conditions should take Vitamin E.

Minerals

1/. Calcium - Calcium supplements can reduce many symptoms of PMS by as much as 30%. Calcium supplements are often poorly absorbed especially inorganic sources such as dolomite. Calcium should be combined with magnesium in the ratio of 2 to 1. A supplement should ideally contain other minerals and vitamins needed in the right proportions. Calcium taken alone depletes zinc and iron. Try a supplement that goes something like this 1000mg calcium,500mg magnesium, 5 mg zinc, with also a little bit of boron. Also take about 1000mg of vitamin C daily.

2/. Chromium - Helps to improve efficient use of insulin and keep blood sugar levels steady. Take 100 to 200 micrograms once or twice a day.

Food Sources - Asparagus, grape juice, prunes, raisins, nuts, mushrooms, molasses.

3/. Magnesium - Alleviates the irritability, fatigue, depression and edema of PMS. This mineral is often deficient in women who consume a diet that is high in refined carbohydrates and sugar. Such diets deplete the body of the minerals chromium, manganese, zinc , magnesium and the B complex vitamins. Women with PMS have been found to have lower levels of magnesium in their red blood cells compared to unaffected women. Women with magnesium deficiency often crave sugar and in particular chocolate. Magnesium is a very important mineral for the nervous system and a deficiency can cause cramps.

Food sources - lettuce, garlic, tomatoes, potatoes, raisins, bananas, almonds, cashews, dates, most whole grains, wheat germ, spinach, peas, celery.

4/. Zinc - Commonly deficient in the western diet. Zinc is necessary for the proper functioning of the ovaries and the reproductive system in both sexes and is also needed for the immune system. It promotes strong and healthy skin and hair and helps in wound healing.

Food sources - Rose hip tea, brewer's yeast, wheat germ, pumpkin seeds, egg yolk and oysters, now you know why oysters are meant to be a aphrodisiac.

Amino Acids

1/. Tryptophan (Amino Acid) - Women with flushes and night sweats can have their symptoms relieved by taking 500mg in fruit juice before sleep. Tryptophan has been found to significantly reduce premenstrual irritability, tension, mood swings, fluid retention breast tenderness and headaches because the body converts it to serotonin. The types of depression that can be treated with Tryptophan are usually associated with cravings for carbohydrates.

Food sources - Cottage cheese, soybean, fish, lintels,

peanuts, pumpkin seeds, sesame seeds.

2/. Glutamine (Amino Acid) - Helps to improve mental clarity, fatigue, reduces blood sugar, reduces sugar cravings, alleviates aggressiveness, improves mood, improves concentration and lifts depression. Take 500 to 1000mg twice daily for 3 months.

Food Sources - Papaya, celery, parsley, spinach, cabbage, lettuce, carrots and Brussels sprouts.

3/. Tyrosine (Amino Acid) - Alleviates the headache, anxiety, fatigue and depression experienced by many females with PMS.

Others

Evening Primrose Oil - This is the most important supplement out of the lot. A lot of people have found that just taking this and B6 can get rid of their problems. EPO (Evening Primrose Oil) is an essential fatty acid and here we are using it to balance the prostaglandin families. What we are trying to do is replace the bad fats with the good ones. EPO increases the good prostaglandins and can be remarkably effective in reducing premenstrual headaches, arthritis, breast tenderness, period pains and other symptoms of PMS. EPO is helpful for ovarian function and helps to return regularity to the menstrual cycle and can also reduce ovarian cysts and ease any pains and inflammations. Try taking about 3 x 1000mlg oil capsules a day. Sometimes you have to take this for a few months to gain the full benefit.

Acidophilus Bacteria - Normalizes the Bowel Flora and helps decrease the reabsorption of estrogens.

Notes

Diet

Nutritional Faults Common In PMS Sufferers

1/. A high blood level of estrogen can be caused by over production, from the diet indirectly by producing too much fat as fat in women makes estrogen, or by decreased break down by the liver. High estrogen levels are associated with deficiencies of the Vitamin B complexes, especially B6 and B12. The liver requires these vitamins to break down and deactivate estrogen.

2/. A high consumption of dairy products. (Dairy animals are feed or injected with artificial hormones).

3/. Excessive consumption of caffeine in the form of soft drinks, coffee and chocolate.

4/. Excessive consumption of refined sugar and not enough whole grains and vegetables.

5/. Excessive consumption of animal fat which leads to the increased levels of the hormone Prostaglandin 2 and also contributes to excess estrogen/low progesterone levels in PMS.

6/. Prostaglandin 2 is a well-known nasty because it increases pain and inflammation and also makes the blood platelets sticky which is its main claim to fame for this is what causes heart attacks and strokes for sticky platelets like blocking off blood vessels. The main source of these as mentioned is animal fats, full cream dairy products, fried foods and takeaways.

7/. Excess body weight is a common factor in PMS

8/. Low levels of Vitamin C and E and Selenium. As with the B vitamins the liver requires these substances to metabolize estrogen properly.

9/. A deficiency in magnesium. Chocolate cravings have been linked to low magnesium levels. Also alcohol and caffeine have been shown to increase urinary excretion of magnesium. High levels of fat in the intestines can interfere with the absorption of magnesium and the liver needs it to.

10/. Light is a nutrient to. Women with PMS exposed to 2 hours of natural light had improvement in their symptoms. This is not as silly as it sounds because you need sunlight to make Vitamin D and you need vitamin D to make calcium.

Diet And Nutrition

I had to give this topic a bit of thought as Diet and Nutrition is such a complex subject that can get very confusing so I have decided that the best way to present this is to keep it as simple as possible. Above we have shown you what the nutrition is like for those women who have PMS. It now looks like the best diet is a kind of diabetes and heart diet combined. In other words a complex carbohydrate diet (low GI) with very low animal fat. Below is the GI index. Here are other factors to consider in making yourself a suitable diet.

1/. Increase Fiber to remove excess estrogens from the

body and improve bowel function.

2/. Add to the diet Phytohormones especially Isoflavones so these natural hormones may buffer the effects of the nasty ones.

3/. Try to eliminate the Faulty Nutrition Common to most PMS sufferers.

4/. Look at the Acid and Alkaline chart for it is said disease cannot live in an Alkaline body. Refined sugar breaks down to acid in the body,.so a low GI diet is actually making your body more alkaline.

5/. Doing all the above is virtually a change of lifestyle so sit down and think about it very carefully and try to make something that you can enjoy. Remember change your diet slowly over a period of months not days as the digestive system doesn't like fast changes.

Glycaemic Index

G.I Range: 15 - 50 Enjoy

Brown Pasta, Tortilla, Whole-wheat, Spaghetti, Brown Rice, Most fruits, Dried Apricots, Dried Apples, Fruit Juices (best diluted with 50% water), Beans, Lentils, Pulses, Peas, High bran cereals, porridge, Most Vegetables, Dairy Foods, Fructose sugar, FOS Sugar.

G.I Range: 50 - 70 Limit

Watermelon, Bananas, Potatoes with skin, Muesli, many plain biscuits, Rye Crisp Bread, Wholemeal Bread, Oatcakes, Most Dried Fruit, Jam.

G.I Range: 79 - 100 Avoid

Glucose, Maltose, Sugar, White Bread, White Rice, Rice Cakes, Cornflakes, Rice Puffs, Cooked Parsnips and Carrots, French Fries, Mashed Potatoes, Water Crackers, Soft Drinks, Sweet Biscuits, Alcohol

Diet For PMS

Well after reading the faults common in PMS some of the things you have to do are fairly obvious. Probably the first and most important one is to get down to your right weight.

1/.Have a high complex carbohydrate low fat diet. Complex carbohydrates are what their name implies they are complex so it takes a while to break down in digestion and this is good because it is releasing the sugars slowly which is what we want. Refined carbohydrates release their sugars fast which leads to high blood sugar then usually follows a slump of low blood sugar (hypoglycaemia) and we all know high blood sugar causes diabetes. Always add a little bit of protein as this makes the complex carbohydrates more complex when all mixed up in the tummy and slows down digestion. Remember busy tummies don't complain for more.

2/. Elimination of refined sugar and refined flower products. Yes I know it's hard but you are just going to have to go through the artificial sweeteners till you have found one you like. I have not had white sugar now for 5 years ever since my father got diabetes. Refined flours have always been scary to me as we all know you can make glue using flower and water and this is what it does inside of you to as well as being responsible for most of the constipation people suffer from.

Try to use unrefined preferably organic wholegrain products such as wholemeal bread, wholemeal flour for cakes, biscuits etc., whole meal pasta, and brown rice.

3/. Elimination of Caffeine - well at least give it a go. I am down to 1 cup of coffee a day now. One of the problems here is that normally there is a lot of sugar with these products so cutting down in one helps with the other. Caffeine in some can bring on panic attacks. One of the big problems today is the high caffeine, high sugar energy drinks. These have now changed society especially for the police who now deal with drunks on these drinks who don't drop off to sleep like they used to but want to fight all the way. I remember recently while working in a chemist in the city a Doctor telling me of a young teenage girl who collapsed in the Mall after drinking 13 cans and later died in hospital.

4/. Increase intake of green leafy vegetables to boost dietary fiber (and magnesium to) and promote hormone clearance. Eat as much as possible of your fruits and vegies raw.

5/. Reduce salt intake, use vegetable salt instead of the normal table salt. If you suffer from fluid retention don't have any salt at all for the week after ovulation.

6/. Increase vegetable protein intake (nuts, beans and pulses including Soya products).

7/. If you are trying to lose weight have some protein with every meal. As mentioned before complex carbohydrates take a while for the digestive system to break down and protein is a lot more complex. This mixture should ensure that tummy is kept busy for a while and not asking for more.

8/. Increase consumption of essential fatty acids, dietary sources are found in raw nuts and seeds. Our Evening Primrose oil Supplement should cover most of this but see what you can do with the diet.

9/. Reduce your stress levels and start some form of exercise even if it's just a walk on the beach.

10/. Don't be too hard on your selves, give yourself your favorite meal on each 7th day and don't nag at yourself to much if you let yourself down just get up again and carry on the path.

If you follow a diet like this for life you would probably slowly reduce in weight, would reduce your chances of heart problems later in life, protect yourself from diabetes, have a good trouble free digestive system and be a very healthy person. If you get the acid and alkaline balance right you could also avoid cancers and chronic disease.

Phytohormones

This can sometimes help with PMS. To quickly explain before you read on what we are trying to do is replace some of your hormones with plant hormones that fit the chemical receptors but have little action on them. So we are in essence trying to buffer the effects of your and any of the rogue ones you have in your body from pollution (pesticides) or from processed food especially Dairy which uses lots of artificial hormones. This gives you another option to try and experiment with.

Some plants are good sources of certain compounds which are capable of moderating our own hormones. These compounds have been dubbed Phytohormones. Phyto means plants and plants can be sources of both Phytoestrogen and Phyto-progesterones. In the last decade there has been particular interest in Phytoestrogens which have the ability to balance our hormones.

Estrogens travel through the body by the blood circulation which takes them eventually to the sites they seek where they bind with the hormone receptor sites which are a bit like a docking terminal which the hormones can lock into and carry out their business. If the hormones that lock into this site are strong or damaging estrogens (from pesticides), they send out magnified messages to the cells to behave in a particular way. This may influence tissues to speed up growth and become more swollen resulting maybe in swollen breasts, lumps, fibroids and endometrial cancers.

Phytoestrogens are remarkable because they can also lock onto these receptor sites and have an effect on them which is much gentler then either our naturally produced estrogens or the xenoestrogens to which we are exposed to from the environment. When Phytoestrogens lock onto the receptor sites their effect is 100 to 1000 times weaker than other sources of estrogens. Not only is their effect weaker but more importantly they block the receptor site from use by other estrogens so this action alone can buffer the system form extreme attacks of unbalanced hormones and also protect you against the negative effects of damaging estrogens.

These Phytoestrogens also have another remarkable health benefit when our own levels of estrogen diminish on the approach of menopause they can act as a hormone replacement. There is now strong research showing that Phytoestrogens from foods and herbs have a positive effect on the early effects of menopause such as hot flushes and vaginal dryness as well as the longer term potential problems such as cardiovascular disease, osteoporosis and breast cancer.

There are around 300 known sources of Phytoestrogens. The most potent sources from foods are Soya products, linseeds, whole-wheat, rye and chickpeas. The Phytoestrogens in Soya foods are called **Isoflavones** and have been the subject of intense study in recent years particularly in their hormone moderating effects which influence menopausal symptoms.

Isoflavones attracted interest because Asian women especially Japanese had lower incidences of breast cancer and have no words for hot flushes in their language and from this further research has suggested Isoflavones in Soya may have a significant effect on preventing the incidence of hormonal problems.

Before embarking on regimes of taking herbs or even

natural hormones it is wise to start increasing the levels of Soya foods and other Phytoestrogen rich food in your diet. Remember your body doesn't like fast changes being made to its diet and will probably complain if this is done so make your changes slowly but surely over a period of a few months.

Sources Of Phytoestrogens

1/. Soya Foods: Soya beans, soya flour, soya flakes, soya mince, soya yoghurt, soya milk, tofu, tempeh and miso.

2/. Whole Grains: Brown rice, whole wheat, barley, rye, millet, corn, buckwheat.

3/. Legumes: Chick peas, peas, peanuts, lentils, lima beans, mung beans, pinto beans.

4/. Seeds and Nuts: Sunflower seeds, sesame seeds, linseeds (Flax seeds), almonds.

5/. Vegetables and Fruit: Fennel, celery, parsley, green beans, sprouted beans, grains, seeds, seaweed, spinach, mushrooms, rhubarb, apples, grapes, citrus fruit.

Phytoestrogen / Isoflavone Levels Of Soya Food

Soya Flakes - half cup = 130mg

Soya Flower - half cup = 85mg

TVP (Soya mince) - half cup = 70mg

Soya Beans Cooked - 100gms = 35mg

Soya Beans Sprouted - 100gms = 35mg

Tempeh - half cup = 35mg

Tofu (full fat) - 100gms = 30mg
Tofu (low Fat) - 100gms = 20mg
Soya Yoghurt - 100gms = 15mg
Soya milk (full Fat) - 1 cup = 10mg
Soya Milk (low fat) - 1cup = 5mg
Miso - 1 tbs = 5mg
Soya Cheese - 100mg = 3mg
  These Can Also Be Brought In Supplement
Form Look For Isoflavones

Nutrition For The Reproductive System

The 5 star Super Foods

Seeds especially pumpkin and sesame
Oats
Avocado
Walnuts
Extra Virgin Olive Oil
Celery
Bananas

The Super Foods

Fruits - Dates. pineapple, citrus fruits, cherries
,blackcurrants, strawberries, rosehips, olives, apricots,

peaches.

Vegetables - Carrots, dark green vegetables, onions, avocado, nettles.

Grains - Maze, oats, whole wheat bread, wheat germ, buckwheat, millet, rye flower.

Pulses - Soybeans, lentils, peas, beans.

Nuts and Seeds - Alfalfa, sprouted seeds, mung beans, soy beans, almonds, hazelnuts, peanuts, cashew nuts.

Herbs and Spices - Parsley, peppermint, fenugreek, sage.

Others - Cold pressed sunflower oil, oily fish, cod liver oil, cheeses, butter, brewer's yeast, molasses, honey, pollen eggs, oysters and shellfish.

The Danger Foods

Fats - In excess, old and rancid fats or foods cooked in them.

Refined Carbohydrates - White flour and sugar deplete levels of B vitamins they are also a heavy tax on the digestive system which drains vital energy. Avoid processed foods.

Meat - Choose organic and free range meat and poultry to avoid the possible ingestion of chemicals from animal medicines and treated animal feed. Sea food is good.

Tonic Herbs For This System - Female - Black haw, Damiana, Dong Quai, Siberian Ginseng, Squaw vine, Liquorices.

An Excess Acid Diet And PMS

An excessively acid diet is one that has lots of protein, sugar, artificial sweeteners and stress which also raises the acid levels of the body. The diet should be about 60% alkaline to 40% acid. It is said that disease can't live in alkaline body. See if you can download an Acid and Alkaline Chart. I feel it's best to start here before we get into the Diet for PMS because if you are living in the Acid Lane then this must be changed as well. This gives you a chance to go through the foods and find the ones that you like. Getting this right now will; save you from problems in the future and may even help you now for it will be taking a load off the body and allowing it to do what it should be doing.

Introducing the Acid and Alkaline Chart

I now believe one of the main causes of cancer is from the body being constantly acidic. It is said **Disease and Cancer are found in Acid bodies, it is said Cancer can't live in an alkaline body.** My training as an Iridologist taught me to see what acid eyes look like and the constant contacts of people with cancer over the years slowly lead me to this conclusion. So a long time ago I made my own Acid and Alkaline Chart as it was the only way I could get one at the time. For over a decade everyone with cancer was shown the chart and we tried to work out where their diet was and nearly all the time they were in the acid areas of the chart or as I refer to it in the acid lane or living in the acid lane. . Recently I was in a very large Pharmacy in the middle of a state capital city for a few years where I had dealings with literally thousands of people with lots of them being tourists. Anyone with cancer was shown the chart and had it explained to them with the result of most of them being in the acid lane not only in food but usually from stress, worry and overwork. Anger also raises the acid levels and I have seen many who are angry and now even more angry that their body has betrayed them and who's going to look after my young family now. They stand in front of me with their fists clenched tight and you can almost feel the rage, this is not fair, it's not right, what am I going to do, who will look after my family. Using this as an example you can see why you have to remove the cause. You have to explain to them what their rage and diet is doing to them. Someone with that amount of anger and stress is rapidly using up all their B vitamins along with calcium and magnesium which the nervous system would be gobbling up at a fast rate as its taking most of the burden from the stress and then imagine how much adrenaline must be in the blood of one so angry so that's more B vitamins are being used to support that system. Let's move this case further along and see what else is happening. Human blood is always slightly alkaline if it goes into the acid we die of what is called Acidosis. So if you are living in the acid lane and your blood is in a constant battle to keep itself in the alkaline lane then the body is in constant stress which makes more acid, but it has no choice but to keep it self-alkaline so to do that it has to use the minerals in the body to buffer that acid with the main ones being Calcium and Magnesium. So imagine a lifetime in the acid lane living on processed food and fizzy drinks which are pumped full of carbonic acid to make the bubbles and loaded with sugar which breaks down to acid and you get the sad picture of lots of people with cancer and lots of people with osteoporosis because the blood has had to steal its Calcium and Magnesium from the bones because it's taken it from every other place as much as it can without breaking down the system. Sometimes the chemist has sent over to me people with cancer who are obviously close to the end of their time and I have shown them the chart, explained it and then given them a photocopy of it and a couple of months later they will pop up and come and see me and say they think it has helped them a bit.

Guide To The Chart

Excessively acid bodies try to make themselves more Alkaline so they tend to use what is easily available to do this which is usually Calcium and Magnesium which do a good job of buffering acid. Too much protein puts acid in the system, mainly uric acid which results from the breakdown of protein. Sugar put lots of acid in the body along with alcohol which when you break it down is just sugar. **Disease and Cancer are found in Acid bodies, it is said Cancer can't live in an Alkaline body.** Use alkaline foods to correct the imbalance. This is what the chart is for, it allows you to see if your diet is to acid and it shows you how to change it by eating more alkaline foods and reducing the acid foods.

1/. Human blood pH should be slightly alkaline (7.35 - 7.45). A pH of 7.0 is neutral. A pH below 7.0 is acidic. A pH above 7.0 is alkaline. A blood pH of 6.9, which is only slightly acidic, can induce coma and death.

2/. An acidic pH can occur from an acid forming diet, emotional stress, toxic overload, immune reactions or any process that deprives the cells of oxygen and other nutrients. The body will try to

compensate for acidic pH by using alkaline minerals. If the diet does not contain enough minerals to compensate, a buildup of acids in the cells will occur.

3/. Alkaline or Acid forming describes ash residue after metabolism. Citrus tastes acidic but leaves an alkaline residue.

4/. Disease and Cancer are found in Acid bodies, it is said Cancer can't live in an Alkaline body. Use alkaline foods to correct the imbalance.

5/. Most people eat acid producing processed foods like white flour and sugar and drink acid producing beverages like coffee and soft drinks. We use too many drugs, which are acid forming; and we use artificial sweeteners.

6/. To maintain health, the diet should consist of 60% alkaline forming foods and 40% acid forming foods. To restore health, the diet should consist of 80% alkaline forming foods and 20% acid forming foods.

7/. Generally, alkaline forming foods include: most fruits, green vegetables, peas, beans, lentils, spices, herbs and seasonings, and seeds and nuts.

8/. Generally, acid forming foods include: meat, fish, poultry, eggs, grains, and legumes.

9/. Protein foods combine well with vegetables but not starches. Starches combine well with other vegetables and also light protein such as dairy foods.

10/. Fruit is best on its own. For digestive distress use Lemon juice as this is a great alkalizer.

11/. Try to make the diet 80% alkaline and 20% acid when you start using the chart. Lemon can be added to sauces, casseroles and fish to reduce acid. Nibble on dates etc.

12/. Add lemon juice to the fridge cold water so every time you drink it you are alkalizing the body.

13/. Rest, sleep and exercise are all alkalizers while the negative emotions make acid. Remember to eat according to you occupation.

14/. Deep breathing releases at least 50% of body toxins so set a time aside each day to do this for a while. Remember happy cells don't mutate.

Herbs - Some of the best herbal digestive remedies are Ginger, Peppermint, Chamomile and Dandelion; these can be had in a tea. Apple Cider Vinegar or Lemon can be added to the teas for their alkalizing effect. Foods can be cooked with herbs for those with poor tummies. Think of the mentioned herbs and then add Fennel, Anise, Cayenne, dill, Garlic, Parsley. Fenugreek, Curry etc. See an Herbalist for Herbs more suited to your condition.

The Acid And Alkaline Chart

For protection against Cancer and Osteoporosis use the Acid and Alkaline Chart. Excessively acid bodies try to make themselves more Alkaline so they tend to use what is easily available to do this which is usually Calcium and Magnesium which do a good job of buffering acid. Too much protein puts acid in the system, mainly uric acid which results from the breakdown of protein. Sugar put lots of acid in the body along with alcohol which when you break it down is just sugar. **Disease and Cancer are found in Acid bodies, it is said Cancer can't live in an Alkaline body.** Use alkaline foods to correct the imbalance. This is what the chart is for, it allows you to see if your diet is to acid and it shows you how to change it by eating more alkaline foods and reducing the acid foods. Diet is very important, consider this, every 3 months the blood replaces itself, every year the bones replace themselves. In a year's time are you going to have a healthy body or a junk food body with McDonald bones. Don't forget if you eat on the acid side the bones won't be all that strong anyway.

Extremely Acid Forming Foods - pH 5.0 to 5.5

5.0 - Artificial sweeteners, Overwork, Fear, Stress, Anger, Jealously.

5.5 - Beef, Carbonated soft drinks & fizzy drinks, Cigarettes (tailor made), Drugs, Flour (white, wheat), Goat, Lamb, Pastries & cakes from white flour, Pork, Sugar (white), Beer, Brown sugar, Chicken, Deer, Chocolate, Coffee, Custard with white sugar, Jams, Jellies, Liquor, Pasta (white), Rabbit, Semolina, Table salt refined and iodized, Tea black, Turkey, Wheat bread, White rice, White vinegar (processed).

Moderate Acid - pH 6.0 to 6.5

6.0.-. Cigarette tobacco (roll your own), Fish, Fruit juices with sugar, Maple syrup (processed), Molasses (sulphured), Pickles (commercial), Breads (refined) of corn, oats, rice & rye, Cereals (refined) e.g. Weetabix, corn flakes, Shellfish, Wheat germ, Whole Wheat foods, Wine, Yogurt (sweetened)

6.5 - Bananas (green), Buckwheat, Cheeses (sharp), Corn & rice breads, Egg whole (cooked hard), Ketchup, Mayonnaise, Oats, Pasta (whole grain), Pastry (wholegrain & honey), Peanuts, Potatoes (with no skins), Popcorn (with salt & butter), Rice (basmati), Rice (brown), Soy sauce (commercial), Tapioca, Wheat bread (sprouted organic)

Slightly Acid to Neutral pH 7.0

7.0 - Barley malt syrup, Barley, Bran, Cashews, Cereals, (unrefined with honey-fruit-maple syrup), Cornmeal, Cranberries, Fructose, Honey (pasteurized), Lentils, Macadamias, Maple syrup (unprocessed), Milk (homogenized) and most processed dairy products, Molasses (unsulphered organic), Nutmeg, Mustard, Pistachios, Popcorn & butter, (plain), Rice or wheat crackers (unrefined), Rye,(grain), Rye bread (organic sprouted), Seeds, (pumpkin & sunflower), Walnuts, Blueberries, Brazil nuts, Butter (salted), Cheeses, (mild & crumbly),

Crackers (unrefined rye), Dried beans, Dry coconut, Egg whites, Goats milk (homogenized), Olives (pickled), Pecans, Plums, Prunes.

Slightly Alkaline to Neutral pH 7.0

7.0 – Almonds, Artichokes (Jerusalem), Barley-Malt, Brown Rice Syrup, Brussels Sprouts, Cherries, Coconut (fresh), Cucumbers, Eggplant, Honey (raw), Leeks, Miso, Mushrooms, Okra, Olives ripe, Onions, Pickles, (homemade), Radish, Sea salt, Spices, Taro, Tomatoes, (sweet), Vinegar (sweet brown rice), Water Chestnut, Artichoke (globe), Chestnuts (dry roasted), Egg yolks (soft cooked), Goat's milk and whey (raw), Horseradish, Mayonnaise (homemade), Millet, Olive oil, Rhubarb, Sesame seeds (whole), Soy beans (dry), Soy cheese, Soy milk, Sprouted grains, Tempeh, Tofu, Tomatoes (less sweet), Yeast, (nutritional flakes)

Moderate Alkaline - pH 7.5 to 8.0

8.0 - Apples (sweet), Apricots, Alfalfa sprouts, Arrowroot, Flour, Avocados, Bananas (ripe), Berries, Carrots, Celery, Currants, Dates & figs, (fresh), Garlic, Gooseberry, Grapes (less sweet), Grapefruit, Guavas, Herbs (leafy green), Lettuce, (leafy green), Nectarine, Peaches (sweet), Pears, (less sweet), Peas (fresh sweet), Pumpkin (sweet), Sea salt (vegetable), Spinach

7.5 - Apples (sour), Bamboo shoots, Beans (fresh green), Beets, Bell Pepper, Broccoli, Cabbage; Cauliflower, Carob, Daikon, Ginger (fresh), Grapes (sour), Kale, Lettuce (pale green), Oranges, Parsnip, Peaches (less sweet), Peas (less sweet), Potatoes & skin, Pumpkin (less sweet), Raspberry, Strawberry, Squash, Sweet corn (fresh), Tamari, Turnip, Vinegar (apple cider)

Extremely Alkaline Forming Foods - pH 8.5 to 9.0

8.5 - Agar, Cantaloupe, Cayenne (Capsicum), Dried dates & figs, Kelp, Limes, Mango, Melons, Papaya, Parsley, Seedless grapes, (sweet), Watercress, Seaweeds, Asparagus, Endive, Kiwifruit, Fruit juices, Grapes (sweet), Passion fruit, Pears (sweet), Pineapple, Raisins, Vegetable juices

9.0 – Lemons, Watermelon.

Introduction to Herbal Medicine

Herbal Medicine has been in use and developed continuously since the beginning of time. It mainly evolved from observations from what plants did and the affects they had on people along with their animals. There is also what they call the Doctrine of Signatures which works like this, that flower really looks like an eye, maybe it helps sore eyes? I'll give it a try as my eyes are so sore and red. You know my eye really feels a lot better now, I think I will call that plant Eye Bright (Euphrasia) and tell my friends all about it especially my Dad who gets sore eyes to. In this way hundreds of plants were identified that have a medical action and no doubt there were also a lot of casualties. The next great leap in herbal medicine was the Roman Empire of 2000 years ago. The Great Armies of Rome all had their own Medical Corps with Doctors, Battle Surgeons and Orderlies. It was these men who already had the knowledge of the Greeks that started to put together the best medical manuals in the world while at the same time started developing and using medical instruments and tools some of which are still used today. As the Romans conquered the known world more medicines and knowledge were found and assimilated. The next great leap was modern Chemistry which allowed us to see exactly what herbs were made up of and what parts of the herb causes its medical action. Drug companies have made billions of Dollars from this information as they find the main active ingredient and then make a synthetic version of it, one good example that we all know of is Valium which is the synthetic version of the active ingredient from the herb Valerian. Leaving aside the Drug Companies let's see how Chemistry changed the way that modern herbalists think. Modern science allows us to now know what Actions our herbs perform on the body so we shall carry on using Valerian as a example and see what Medical Actions Valerian has on the body. The Actions of Valerian are Sedative, Hypnotic (sleep inducing), Anti Spasmodic (stops twitches, cramps etc.), Hypotensive (lowers Blood Pressure) and Carminative (calms and relaxes the tummy). Herbalists call Valerian the Herbal Tranquillizer and if you look at the actions you can see why for if you can't sleep and your blood pressures up along with a gurgling tummy and an eye constantly twitching you definitely need to be calmed down. The modern herbalist is trained to think in actions. There are many reasons for this but the main ones are to stop them from just using a handful of their favorite herbs and to train the mind to work in the method of thinking in actions that are needed. If we start thinking in the actions that are needed for a patient it makes us consider the problem in far more depth than just using our favorite herb and it forces our thinking to be far more holistic by taking in consideration the whole of the patient not just the part or the system we wish to treat. Let's take a look at thinking in actions.

The patient has a cough, but when coughs can't stop and the cough sounds a bit like whooping cough. The patient also sounds a little hoarse and the temperature is also elevated. The actions that come into mind for this are expectorant for the cough, antispasmodics for the whooping quality of the cough and demulcents to sooth the sore throat. These are the obvious actions and we can add many more if we wish such as immune boosters for acute diseases, diaphoretics to reduce the temperature and prevent a fever and the list goes on. Next we look at how Herbal Actions are used in making Herbal Formulas. Another point to make before we go to the formula making is that Professional Herbalists use Herbs in the form of Tinctures (water and alcohol solutions) as this allows them to mix formulas in any proportions that they like and also allows long term storage without spoiling.

Making Herbal Formulas

You should never have more the 5 Herbs in a herbal formula otherwise you start to lose track of what you are doing and how the formula is changing the symptoms. Always try to keep things simple. One of the herbs in the formula is used to force the formula into the body, to keep it simple we will only use three, they are Licorice, Ginger and Cayenne. As an example let's use a patient with a cough. After further study of the case we decide that this is an Acute Disease for it came on quickly and is fast acting not slow like a

Chronic Disease. Listening to the patients cough we decide that it is a dry cough and the patient has not got a runny nose. Let's list the actions to consider.

Expectorants - Licorice, Aniseed, Fennel, Garlic and Mullein

Antispasmodics - Aniseed and Fennel

Demulcents - Licorice and Coltsfoot

Immune Boosters - Echinacea

Anti-Bacterial and Virals - Garlic and Echinacea

Out of the above I would choose Licorice, Echinacea, Garlic, Aniseed and Fennel. I would make the formula in this strength.

<u>Formula</u>

Licorice - 20%

Garlic - 15%

Echinacea - 15%

Aniseed - 30%

Fennel - 20%

Look these herbs up in the herbal and consider why I used them, there are three obvious ones for Licorice alone with the first being to force the assimilation of the formula into the body, second is its expectorant action and third is its demulcent action in case the throat is sore and raw. Next time you see a little kid eating heaps of licorice get them to open their mouth and look at their tongue which will be going black from the Licorice along with the throat etc. and know that you are looking at the demulcent action of Licorice working by coating and soothing. The most important reason that you use the Actions Method for Herbal Prescribing is so that you can concentrate the Actions which are most needed for example, if it's a Bacterial Infection concentrate on the Anti Bacterials, if it's a Viral infection concentrate on the Anti Virals, hopefully you are now beginning to see the importance of working in actions for if you don't concentrate a large part of the battle on the causes you may have lost the battle from the start. Read through all the Actions listed in Herbal Actions in the book and then do a study in depth of at least five Actions of your choice making the first two the Anti Bacterials and Anti Virals. Start trying to train your mind into thinking in Actions.

\

How To Make Herbal Tinctures

Tinctures are made by steeping the Herb plant material in a mixture of alcohol and water. Alcohol is usually always used at strength of 45%. The alcohol in this mixture will extract all the essential oils from the herb while the water will extract all that is water soluble, so between the both we are getting most of the medicinal properties out of the herb. The proportions of herb to liquid are usually 1 part herb to 5 parts liquid. So find a suitable container (I use a big one liter preserving jar with a good sealing lid) and put into it 100grams of your chosen herb and to that add 500mls of our 45% solution of alcohol. Seal the lid and shake well for about a minute. Leave the jar on the window sill so the sun can shine on the jar for two weeks. The jar must be shaken for at least a minute every day. After 2 weeks open and filter the contents of the jar. I use a large pouring jug into which I place a funnel and then place a coffee filter in the funnel and pour the jar contents through the funnel being careful not to let too much herb spill into the filter and block it up. When you get to the bottom of the jar you can crush the herb in your fist so as to extract the last of the liquid. After this is completed you then get your chosen storage bottle, put a funnel into its neck followed by a coffee filter and then filter the jug into the bottle. Remember the solution should always be double filtered Next we label the bottle, put the date, name and proportions e.g. 1 to 5 also state the recommended dose. Store in a cool and dark place. Most Professional Homoeopaths and Herbalists have access to pure alcohol so for them it is fairly easy to make tinctures while for the lay person they will probably have a hard time. An alternative is to use Vodka as strong as you can find it or find a way to twist the authorities arm into giving alcohol at 45%. Don't even try to get pure alcohol as it is dangerous and can turn people blind and they won't give it to you.

How To Make Infusions

Infusions are a bit like making a cup of tea except we don't use milk. Infusions are used for the soft parts of the herb such as the flowers, leaves and fine twigs. The proportions for infusions are 1 to 20 e.g. 1 part herb to 20 parts water. Infusions are used for the more water soluble herbs. Infusions can be made from a single herb or from a combination of herbs and may be drunk hot or cold. The water should be just off the boil before being poured on the herb and if you are making an infusion of a herb strong in essential oils such as Peppermint always cover the top of the cup to stop the essential oils from escaping in steam while the infusion is brewing. Allow up to 10 minutes to brew. It is best to make herbal teas fresh each day. You can experiment on yourself by getting

Chamomile and Peppermint tea bags from the supermarket. Use honey as a sweetener.

How To Make Decoctions

Decoctions are used for the more hard woody substances of the herb such as barks, berries or roots. The process of decoction is far more vigorous then infusion as it involves heating the plant material in cold water, bringing it to the boil and simmering for 20 to 40 minutes. The finished ratio for decoctions is again 1 part herb to 20 parts water; remember to add more water at the beginning so you wind up with the 1 to 20 after steam loss. This form of preparation is no good for the herbs that are high in essential oils as these will all be lost in the steam.

Glossary of Herbal Terms And Index Of Actions

Adaptogen - Helps the body overcome its problems and work to the best of its ability. Good convalescent herbs.

Herbs - Panax Ginseng, Siberian Ginseng .Schizandra, Withania.

Alterative - Herbs that gradually restore proper function to the body, they increase health and vitality. They were once known as the blood cleansers.

Herbs - Beth root, Black cohosh, Damiana, Dong Quai , Red Clover, Sarsaparilla, Skullcap.

Analgesic - Herbs that reduce pain.

Herbs - Black Haw, Chamomile, Dong Quai, Hops, Ladys Mantle, Passion Flower, St Johns Wort, Skullcap, Valerian, Wild Yam, Withania.

Antidepressive - Damiana, Rosemary, Skullcap , St Johns Wort, Valerian, Vervain.

Anti-fungal - Calendula, Cats Claw, Pau D' Arco, Myrrh, Olive Leaf.

Anti-inflammatory - Helps the body to combat inflammations. Herbs mentioned under demulcents, emollients and vulnerary's will often act in this way especially when they are applied externally.

Herbs - Black Cohosh, Blue Cohosh, Chamomile, Feverfew, Ginger, Ladys Mantle, St Johns Wort, Sage, Wild Yam, Withania.

Anti-microbial - Helps the body destroy or resist

pathogenic micro-organisms.

Herbs - Aniseed, Rosemary, Sage, Thyme Yarrow

Anti-oxidant - Milk Thistle, Schizandra.

Antispasmodic - Prevents or eases spasms and cramps.

Herbs - Aniseed, Angelica, Black Haw, Beth root, Black cohosh, Blue Cohosh, Chamomile, Cramp Bark, Dong Quai, Hops, Motherwort, Passion Flower, Red Clover, Rosemary, Sage, Skullcap, St johns Wort, Valerian, Vervain, Wild Yam.

Anti-viral - St Johns Wort

Antirheumatic - Black cohosh, blue cohosh, dandelion, sarsaparilla,

Aperient - Mild laxative.

Herbs -Dandelion, Fenugreek, Milk Thistle.

Astringent - Contracts tissue which in turn reduces discharges, these herbs contain tannins.

Herbs - Black Haw, Beth root, Hops, Ladys Mantle, Sage, raspberry, Rosemary, Squaw Vine, Shepherds Purse, St Johns Wort, Yarrow.

Bitter - Herbs that taste bitter act as stimulating tonics for the digestive system.

Herbs - Feverfew, Hops,

Carminative - Stimulates peristalsis of the digestive system and relaxes the stomach and helps remove gas and wind from the system. These herbs are usually rich in volatile oils.

Herbs - Aniseed, angelica, chamomile, garlic, ginger, sage, rosemary, valerian.

Cardioactive - Has a effect on the heart.

Herbs - Motherwort,

Circulatory Stimulant - Siberian Ginseng, ginger, rosemary

Cholagogue - Stimulates the release of bile from the gallbladder which can relieve gallbladder problems, bile is also the body's natural laxative so cholagogues have a laxative effect as well.

Herbs - Dandelion, milk thistle.

Demulcent - Soothes and protects irritated or inflamed internal tissues.

Herbs - fenugreek, licorice, milk thistle, sarsaparilla

Diaphoretic - Aids the skin in the elimination of toxins and produces sweat thus reducing the temperature of fevers.

Herbs - Angelica, black cohosh, chamomile, garlic, ginger, sarsaparilla, thyme, vervain, yarrow.

Diuretic - Increases the secretion and elimination of urine.

Herbs - Agrimony, angelica, dandelion leaves, false unicorn root, ladys mantle, shepherds purse, red clover, sarsaparilla, yarrow.

Emmenagogue - Stimulates and normalizes the menstrual flow, tonics for the female reproductive system.

Herbs - Angelica, black cohosh, blue cosh, chamomile, cramp bark, dong quai, false unicorn root, fenugreek, ginger, ladys mantle, motherwort, raspberry, sage, rosemary, shepherds purse, St Johns

Wort, thyme, Valerian, vervain, yarrow.

Expectorant - Supports the body in the removal of excess mucous from the respiratory system and helps in the control of coughs.

Herbs -Angelica, aniseed, fenugreek, garlic, red clover, thyme, vervain.

Febrifuge - Helps the body to bring down fevers.

Herbs - Raspberry, sage, thyme, vervain.

Galactagogue - Helps increase the flow of milk in females.

Herbs - Aniseed, fenugreek, milk thistle, raspberry, vervain.

Hepatic - Tones and strengthens the liver, may increase the flow of bile.

Herbs - Agrimony, dandelion, motherwort, milk thistle, vervain, yarrow.

Hormone Precursors - Provide the building blocks for hormones.

Herbs - Beth root, Black Cohosh, Blue Cohosh, Licorice, Fenugreek, Ginseng, Sarsparillia, Wild Yam, Withania

Infusion - Is like how you make a cup of tea but when you make herb teas you don't use milk. Pour boiling water onto the herb in the cup and cover the cup (to stop the essential oils from evaporating) and leave for about 5 minutes. To sweeten add honey.

Laxative - Promotes the evacuation of the bowels.

Herbs - Dandelion, fenugreek,

Lotion - A water and tincture mixture, example 2 parts tincture to 20 parts water.

Nervine - Has a beneficial effect on the nervous system, acts like a tonic to this system.

Herbs - Black cohosh, blue cohosh, chamomile, cramp bark, damiana, hops, motherwort, oats, rosemary, skullcap, St Johns Wort, schizandra, thyme, valerian, vervain.

Parasiticide - Kills parasites and insects.

Herbs - Aniseed, rosemary.

Pectoral - Has a general strengthening and healing effect on the respiratory system.

Herbs - Aniseed, garlic, hyssop, vervain.

Sedative - Calms the nervous system and reduces stress and nervousness throughout the body.

Herbs - Black Haw, Black cohosh, chamomile, cramp bark, hops, motherwort, passion flower, skullcap, St Johns Wort, schizandra, valerian, vervain.

Stimulants - Quicken and enliven the physiological function of the body.

Herbs - Dandelion, garlic, rosemary, sage, yarrow.

Tincture - Herbal tinctures are made from herbs mixed with a water and alcohol mix of about half and half and are usually of the strength of 1 part herb to 5 parts solvent.

Tonics - Strengthen and enliven specific organs or the whole body.

Herbs - Aniseed, Beth root, black cohosh, blue cohosh, chamomile, dandelion, fenugreek, motherwort, oats, raspberry, sarsaparilla, skullcap, thyme, vervain, yarrow.

Urinary Antiseptic - Angelica, damiana, shepherds purse, yarrow

Vasodilator - Black cohosh, Dong quai, feverfew, ginger, yarrow

Herbs Used For Female Problems

Below are listed some of the main herbs for Female Problems that Herbalists use. Herbalists never prescribe for just the disease alone but always prescribe on an individual basis because the reality is that there is just about as many different forms of disease as there are people who have it. Some of the herbs listed below may be hard for you to find but most Health Shops should be able to get them and there are now lots of good Herbal suppliers on the internet now.

With Herbal treatment it is best to get this done professionally especially in complex matters, making sure of course that you bring along your chart with you. The reason for this is that an herbalist will treat you holistically and not just the most bothersome symptoms. This is very important and the best way to show you is to give you an example of how I might treat someone with PMS problems.

When I make a Herbal formula which is usually in tincture form I try to use no more than 5 herbs, and for a women with PMS problems one herb would go to help and support the liver whose job is to keep the hormones at the right levels and to disassemble the excess, while the remaining herbs would go to helping the main symptoms of the case. With these I would try to choose herbs that could be converted into hormones easily so they could act in two ways at the same time with one being to target the problem symptoms and the other being to increase the phytoestrogens in the body so as to increase the binding of hormone receptor sites with phytoestrogens instead of the bodies more powerful estrogens and in this way I may be able to buffer the hormone reactions which may in turn lessen the problem symptoms. So as you can now see there is a lot more that goes into it then just prescribing herbs for the symptoms.

For most people reading this you will probably make your combination of herbs in teas. As this book has been designed for people in the country away from easily accessible Medical Treatment I will go into detail about selecting and individualizing a herbal formula suitable for yourself.

The best way to start is to sit down and write out your main symptoms or the ones most annoying to you in order of their importance but do not go over about 8 strong symptoms for the idea is to try and keep this reasonably easy. As you have read before we try to use only 5 herbs in the formula with one being for the liver and another from our list of Hormone Precursors in the Herbal Actions List. The last 3 herbs along with the first 2 should cover most of our symptoms and for the strong symptoms we want at least the actions of 2 herbs to cover that symptom so as to enhance the action in that area. A good example is below. This women's PMS is now being complicated by the onset of menopause.

Example Patient 1

Here we have a woman just at the onset of menopause that has always had PMS problems. She is also getting rheumatism beginning in her fingers and back which most of the women in her family get starting at her age. She is just beginning to get her first Hot Flashes and is getting depressed and moody and also having trouble sleeping.

Formula

Black Cohosh
Dandelion
Sage
Skullcap
Passion Flower

Black Cohosh – Is a Hormone Precursor and also one of the main hormones balancers especially for the onset of menopause. The herb is also used for pains, especially those of Rheumatism and in our patients case we are also using it for sleep. This will be our main remedy in the formula given at strength stronger than all the others.

Dandelion – Is a good liver herb given for reasons already mentioned but where there is depression also consider looking at the liver especially when there is anger with it. Dandelion is also important for PMS.(B) as the leaf of this herb is one of our main diuretics which removes fluid from the body. Dandelion is the safest diuretic you can use because it puts more potassium into the body then what its diuretic action takes out. So when using diuretics always be careful not to take out excess potassium.

Sage - Covers the Hot Flashes for which it is a specific and probable sweating.

Skullcap - Covers depression, insomnia and moods and works with the nervous system calming the system.

Passion Flower -.Covers insomnia, moods and touches on the depression and could help with the pains of rheumatism.

The above is a good example of overlapping Actions of Herbs while at the same time having our Liver Herb and Hormone Precursor Herb.

Example Patient 2

This Lady has just turned 24 and thinks she has always had PMS problems but they have now got a lot worse since she has started a new job and is now under constant stress and has to perform which has brought on anxiety and panic attacks. Sometimes she can't sleep at night from worrying. Using Iridology and looking at her eyes we can see 3 nerve rings in each eye so she is really stressed. I show her the nerve rings in the mirror and tell her if you get more of them you're getting worse. If you get less, than you're getting better. I pointed out that it's better to remove the cause rather than the end result and we know the cause is stress. She says she will never get an opportunity like this again so she has to go on. We talk for a while and I agree to help her pointing out that she has to adapt to her new role and delegate some work to others if she can so as to reduce the stress and if all fails then it's easier to get a another good job when you've got a good job.

Formula 2

There will be no liver herb in this formula because we know the problem was caused by stress. All stimulants must be stopped especially coffee and the caffeine drinks with one cup of coffee a day so as to help withdrawal symptoms at about 3pm each day. Having the coffee later in the day should hopefully prevent the panic attacks as she should have the day sorted out by then and less to panic about.

Chaste Tree (Vitex Agnus Castus)

Licorice

Withania

Skullcap swapped with Zizyphus later on if still having trouble sleeping.

Chaste Tree – This is the specific for PMS. Chaste Tree acts on the pituitary gland which is the main gland that controls all the hormone glands, so Chaste Tree takes us to the boss.

Licorice – Acts on the adrenal glands which are the main ones that suffer from the effects of stress and helps to restore them to natural function. Adrenal

Tonic. Not for those with Blood Pressure problems.

Withania – Is beginning to be one of the main specifics for stress. Being a Adaptogen it tries to adapt the body to its current situation while its hormone balancing action adds to that of Chaste Tree.

Skullcap – The main action of this herb is on the Central Nervous System which it tries to calm and maintain and is the specific in this area for PMS.

Zizyphus – This herb is kind of the new kid on the block as it has only started being used by western herbalists just recently, and started mainly for sleep with the main company supplying it giving out free samples at the airport. It must have worked as I had lots of customers coming in with their sample pack trying to get it. The Chinese use this herb to calm the mind and cleanse the body. Western Herbalists are using it for sleep and anxiety.

Nutrition - We urgently need to replace the B Vitamins, Calcium and Magnesium as these are what the patient is burning rapidly. The patient has been advised to take a Berocca effervescent B, Cal, Mag and zinc tab in the early morning and at mid-morning a High Strength Multi Vitamin that is very high in the Bs at about 50mg and that has a slow release so all the Bs aren't washed out of the body straight away.

Do Not Use Hormone Balancing Herbs If You Are On The Pill Or Hormone Treatment. Pick on the Adaptogens.

Herbal PMS Formulas

Below is a list of some common Menopause Formulas found usually in boxes at your local Chemist or Health Shop. I will give you the Brand name first followed by the Product Name and then will give you a list of the ingredients. It is now up to you to look up the ingredients in the Herbal and find which product covers most of your symptoms and would be the most suitable for you. A lot of these are not made any more and some of the brands are gone but it gives you an idea of the herbs used in some of the formulas which you can look up and see how they work. Red Clover is a fairly common main ingredient but with this herb all they have done is extracted the estrogens and concentrated them and are not using the herb for its traditional use.

Blackmores

Dong Quai,Vitex Agnus Castus (Chaste Tree)

Ethical Nutrients

Chaste Tree, Zyziphus, B6 and Chromium

Herbs Of Gold

Asparagus, Chaste Tree, B1, B6 and Magnesium

Harmony

Chaste Tree, Dong Quai, Paeonia Lactiflora and Bupleurum Flacatum Root

Nature's Own
Chaste Tree, Black Cohosh and Withania.

Most Others Are Just Repeating What Is Here Especially The Chaste Tree And Magnesium.

Herbal

Aniseed

Actions - Antispasmodic, carminative, expectorant, parasiticide, antimicrobial, galactagogue.

This is a herb with many uses, some of the main uses are intestinal colic and flatulence, a good digestive tonic and appetite stimulant, a good expectorant and along with its antispasmodic action it can be used for such conditions as bronchitis and whooping cough. Aniseed has mild estrogenic effects and can be used as a good herb for relieving some of the symptoms of menopause.

This herb has a reputation of increasing milk production in nursing mothers, promoting menstruation and also facilitating childbirth. It is also said to increase libido in men and women.

Doses - Mainly used as a tea, 1 to 2 teaspoonfuls of seeds add boiling water, cover and leave for 5 to 10 minutes.

Angelica

Actions - Carminative, antispasmodic, expectorant, diuretic, diaphoretic, emmenagogue.

As an expectorant it is good for respiratory infections with coughs accompanied with fever, as a digestive it stimulates appetite and is good for colic and flatulence and this herb may also be used as a urinary antiseptic in cases of cystitis. This herb is a close relation to Dong Quai which is Chinese Angelica and would have similar actions

Doses - Tincture 2 to 5mls 3 times daily, 1 teaspoon full of the cut root in tea 3 times daily.

Astragalus

Actions - Immune-modulator, anti-viral, adaptogen, hypotensive, immune stimulant, adrenal tonic, diuretic, vasodilator, blood tonic.

Stimulates the natural production of interferon (helps to stop viruses replicating) and intensifies the white cell destruction of germs in other words it is a immune booster. A good tonic for strengthening the resistance to disease. Is very useful for people in a state of chronic debility and fatigue by restoring the immune function and giving them energy especially in those with cancer undergoing chemo or people with Ross River Fever this is why the herb is known as a Adaptogen because it helps people adapt and have the energy to cope with changes. Use as a lung tonic to help expel toxins and pus in flu's, colds and sinusitis. Increases stamina and can accelerate wound healing.

Uses - Boosting immune system, disease preventative, fatigue, healing wounds, good for use in those with chronic diseases that cause immune problems such as AIDS.

Beth Root

Actions - Uterine tonic, astringent, expectorant, antispasmodic alterative.

Contains natural precursors of the female sex hormones. Is a tonic for the uterus and its astringent power is used for excessive bleeding or hemorrhage. It is considered a specific for excessive blood loss during menopausal changes. It is mainly used for bleeding due to menses, fibroids and postpartum difficulties.

Black Haw

Actions - Astringent, antispasmodic, sedative, hypotensive, analgesic, uterine tonic.

Has a similar action to cramp bark to which it is closely related. Powerful relaxant of the uterus used for cramps and false labor pains. Can be used to prevent miscarriages. It can relax peripheral blood vessels thus reducing blood pressure. Its use for bleeding is confined to birthing and menopause.

Black Cohosh

Actions - Emmenagogue, anti-spasmodic, nervine, alterative, sedative, tonic, vasodilator.

Black Cohosh has a normalizing action on the balance of female sex hormones and may be safely used to regain normal hormonal activity that should give relief to Menopause and PMS symptoms. This would be the herb for you if you also suffered from rheumatism or arthritis. Has hormone balancing properties, encourages estrogen production, painful or delayed menstruation, ovarian cramps or cramping pain in the womb, used to regain normal hormone activity, good for hot flashes, rheumatoid and osteoarthritis, muscular and neuralgic pains with a good example being Sciatica. Black Cohosh may also lower blood pressure, lower cholesterol, help with insomnia and help with tinnitus.

Doses - For tincture is 2-4mls 3 times a day, One and a half teaspoonful's for tea 3 times a day.

Cautions - Best taken with meals so as to avoid any chance of upsetting tummy. Allow up to 8 weeks to see benefits in menopausal problems and even then the full benefit of the herb may not be reached till 6 month's time. Antibiotics can reduce the effect of this herb. This herb can interfere with hormonal medications eg The Pill. Contra indicated in pregnancy.

Blue Cohosh

Actions - Nervine, antispasmodic, uterine tonic, diuretic, emmenagogue, antirheumatic.

As a emmenagogue this herb can be used to bring on delayed or suppressed menstruation while ensuring that the pain sometimes accompanied is relieved. Good for most pains and spasms associated with the menstrual cycle and reproductive organs. Can be used for leucorrhoea and vaginitis. Blue Cohosh may be used where there is a need for a antispasmodic such as in colic, asthma and nervous coughs and it also has a good reputation for easing rheumatic pain.

Doses - Tincture 1 to 2mls 3 times daily, 1 teaspoon of dried root for tea 3 times a day.

Caution - Can further increase blood pressure in people with high blood pressure.

Chamomile

Actions - Antispasmodic, nervine, carminative, anti-inflammatory, analgesic, antiseptic, allergies.

An excellent gentle sedative with a relaxing action that is good for easing anxiety and helping with sleep. In the digestive system it can be used for indigestion especially when there is colicky pains and is ideal for colitis and IBS type problems. For females Chamomile is good for amenorrhea, spasmodic dysmenorrhea, premenstrual irritability and menopausal tensions. This herb is also a good source of calcium and magnesium.

Doses - Tincture 2 to 4mls 3 times daily, for teas just the one teabag.

Cramp Bark

Actions - Nervine, sedative, astringent, antispasmodic, tonic, emmenagogue, dysmenorrhea.

As the name suggests this herb is a relaxer of muscular tension and spasms. It has to main areas of use with the first being muscular cramps and the second in ovarian and uterine muscle problems. Cramp Bark relaxes the uterus and relieves spasms and cramps and can be used to help prevent a miscarriage. This herb also has a astringent action which gives it a role in the treatment of excessive blood loss in periods and especially bleeding associated with menopause.

Doses - Tincture 4 to 8mls 3 times a day, for tea 2 teaspoonful's of the dried bark 3 times a day.

Dandelion

Actions - Diuretic, cholagogue, antirheumatic, laxative, tonic.

Here we will mainly be using Dandelion for its diuretic action so as to ease fluid retention.

For this it is best to use the leaf. Dandelion is a gentle and safe diuretic because unlike others it actually gives the body more potassium then it takes out.

Doses - Tincture 5 to 10mls 3 times daily, 2 to 3 teaspoons of herb for tea 3 times daily.

Damiana

Actions - Nerve Tonic, antidepressant (sexual matters), urinary antiseptic, alterative, reproductive tonic.

A good herb for strengthening the nervous system and it also has a tonic action on the hormonal system. Considered to be a specific in cases of anxiety and depression where there is a sexual factor. Damiana may help to reduce hot flashes and may increase sex drive and can be used for cystitis, headaches and insomnia.

Doses - Tincture 1 to 2mls 3 times daily, 1 teaspoon of dried leaves 3 times daily.

Note - Longer use of Damiana increases its potency and helps to regulate sex hormones in women but it may also interfere with iron absorption.

Dong Quai see also Angelica

Actions - Emmenagogue, antispasmodic, analgesic, alterative, uterine tonic ,vasodilator.

Relieves some but not all of the symptoms of PMS and menopause by its action as a known regulator for the female reproductive system. Some of its compounds stimulate the uterus while others relax the uterus. The compounds that stimulate the uterus are water soluble and are absorbed into the body from teas and capsules. The compounds that relax the uterus are soluble in alcohol and are provided by tinctures. This herb may stop cramping, migraine attacks and eases the pain of ovarian cysts while there is less agreement on whether the herb stops hot flashes (wait and see after 6 weeks on the herb). The Chinese use this herb for abnormal menstruation, suppressed flow, painful or difficult menstruation. This herb is also good for the treatment of psoriasis. Dong Quai also helps with Anemia related to menses, asthma, bronchitis, emphysema and improves the function of the lungs.

Dose - 6 to 18 grams of dried root per day and in the tablet form 1500mg per day.

Note - This herb has a mild laxative effect. People who take blood thinners should avoid this herb.

Echinacea

Actions - Immune stimulant, anti-microbial, anti-inflammatory, alterative, healing.

Is an infection fighter active against strep bacteria (abscesses and boils), a blood cleanser, (blood poisons, snake bites, poisonous insects) and a glandular and lymphatic system cleanser. Use it particularly for respiration infections and for any disease above the waist. This is one of our main immune boosters for the acute diseases. Use as a prophylactic to protect from infections especially when traveling or before going into Hospital.

Uses - All infections, depressed immune function, inflammatory conditions, allergies, effective against both bacteria and viruses.

Dose – 1 to 4mls of tincture

Warning - Do not use continually as you will burn out the immune system give a few weeks break after 3 weeks. Beware also in the use of allergies for you could be building up the immune system just to attack itself.

False Unicorn Root

Actions - Uterine tonic, emmenagogue, diuretic, emetic, antiseptic, vermafuge.

A tonic that strengthens the reproductive system. Contains estrogen precursors. Useful in delayed or absent menstruation, Good for easing ovarian pain, used as a aid to getting pregnant and staying pregnant as well as for vomiting during pregnancy. Can be used as a restorative tonic after long use of the birth control pill. Can help with physical and emotional wound after sexual abuse and be given to women as a tonic after menopause or hysterectomy.

Feverfew

Actions - Anti-inflammatory, vasodilator, relaxant, digestive bitter, uterine stimulant.

It is one of the most important aids for female ailments with the plant exerting remarkable powers over the uterus. A good treatment for all female irregularities especially scanty or failing menses, painful periods, inflamed or weak uterus, uterine and vaginal ulcers, abortion, difficult labour, retained afterbirth, arthritis, inflammations. May help ease dizziness and tinnitus with other remedies (Black Cohosh). Has a good reputation for migraine headaches, may help with arthritis when it is in the inflammatory stage. This herb may also help with colitis, indigestion, fevers and inflammations.

Dose - Best taken in tablet form. 3x500ml tablets a day.

Fenugreek

Actions - Expectorant, demulcent, tonic, laxative, galactagogue, hypoglycaemic, nutritive.

This herb supports liver function and is protective to the mucous linings of the body as well as having a strong action on the lymphatic system as it clears and promotes the drainage of the body through the lymphatic system. This rubbish removing action can lead to strong body odors and dark urine and maybe even a healing crisis as a life time's load of rubbish starts to get evicted.

This is a good herd to use if you have diabetes. This herb is said to be a good hormone balancer for menopause and may raise estrogen levels.

Doses - Tincture 1 to 2mls 3 times a day, 1 and a half teaspoons of seed (crush seed first to release oils) add boiling water and cover, let stand for 10 minutes. 1 teaspoonful of aniseed can be added to improve the taste. Maybe only use this twice a day and maybe a week on and a week off.

Garlic

Actions - Immune stimulant, anti-bacterial, anti-viral, anti-fungal, anti-septic, anti-oxidant, diaphoretic, cholagogue, hypotensive, anti-spasmodic, vermifuge and many more.

The plant is rich in volatile oil and sulphur and because of its remarkable penetrating, disinfecting and mucous expelling powers garlic is a valuable basic remedy for the treatment of all ailments in which the cleansing of the blood stream and expulsion of mucous accumulations is required. Garlic can be used to prevent and treat respiratory infections. Anyone who has had garlic breath has experienced this herb's aromatic compounds being excreted through their lungs which is why garlic's active ingredients can be so effective for respiratory complaints. Garlic is extremely effective in dissolving and cleansing cholesterol from the blood stream, it stimulates the digestive tract, kills worms, parasites and harmful bacteria, normalizes blood pressure, reduces fever, gas and cramps.

Uses- All infections, coughs, colds, flu, bronchitis, all fevers, pulmonary conditions, gastric and skin complaints, rheumatism, all worms and ringworm, ticks and lice.

Acts on Bacteria, Viruses and Internal Parasites.

Dose – 3000mg Garlic Oil tabs are the best way to go

as tis gets into the blood fast. For those who cannot tolerate the breath use Kyloc the Japanese aged form as this is odourless.

Externally - You can use garlic for ring worm and ear ache, to disinfect wounds and sores, parasitical infections.

Ginger

Actions- Carminative, anti-inflammatory, vasodilator, circulatory stimulant, diaphoretic, anti-emetic.

The therapeutic benefits of ginger are largely due to its volatile oil and oleoresin content. Ginger is an excellent remedy for many digestive complaints, including nausea, colic, wind and indigestion. Its antiseptic properties also make it beneficial for gastro-intestinal infections. It stimulates the circulatory system and helps blood flow and increases stamina. Aids in fighting colds, colitis, digestive disorders, wind, and increases saliva.

Uses- Indigestion, nausea, feverish conditions especially when chills are present, travel sickness especially sea sickness, dyspepsia, colic, flatulence.

Caution - Don't use large doses on an empty stomach..

Ginseng (Panax)

Actions - Anti depressive, stimulating adrenal agent, estrogenic, increases resistance and improves mental and physical performance.

This herb can help with depression especially when caused by debility and exhaustion. It can be used in general for exhaustion and weakness. Used to increase mental and physical performance, to improve concentration, vigilance and work efficiency, stamina, for combating internal or external stress factors of any kind - athletics, endurance activities, aging, surgery, disease, infections, cold, but especially degenerative conditions and problems of old age. This is a god herb for infertility and menopause symptoms.

Doses - For the elderly and long term 400 to 800mgs per day. Short term 600 to 2000mg per day for 3 to 4 weeks then have a break for 4 weeks then you can go back on it if you wish. Remember month on month off as this herb can build up in the system. During your month off you will still be getting the benefits of this herb as the excess leaves the body.

Siberian Ginseng

Actions - Adaptogen, vaso dilator, increases stamina, circulatory stimulant.

This herb is very similar to the one above but is a milder version and can be used all the time without any breaks and does not build up in the system like

Panax Ginseng.

Dose - As what is said on the packet.

Ginger

Actions - Carminative, diaphoretic, circulatory stimulant, sialagogue, vasodilator, antiemetic.

Ginger may be used as a stimulant of the peripheral circulation in cases of bad circulation, chilblains and cramp. In feverish conditions ginger acts as a diaphoretic promoting sweet and cooling the body. As a carminative it promotes gastric secretions and is used in dyspepsia, flatulence and colic. For females ginger can be used for painful menstruation or retarded menstruation. Ginger is good to mix with any other combination of herbs because it would help the body to assimilate those herbs and increase their actions.

Doses - Dose as needed in its various forms.

Hops

Actions - Sedative, hypnotic, bitter, antiseptic, visceral antispasmodic, astringent, estrogenic.

Has a marked relaxing effect on the central nervous system and is used extensively for the treatment of insomnia. Eases tension and anxiety and may be used where this tension leads to restlessness, headaches and indigestion. This is a good herb for Mucous Colitis and colicky types of pain. According to herbal folk law elderly women who worked as hop pickers experienced a return of their menstrual cycles and other youthful attributes. This lead to the use of Hops as a hormone balancer and general restorative during and after menopause. Hops contains the most potent of all the plant estrogens.

Doses - Tincture 1 to 4mls 3 times daily, 1 teaspoon of dried flowers in tea 3 times a day or just before bed.

Ladys Mantle

Actions - Astringent, anti-inflammatory, emmenagogue, diuretic, anodyne, menopause herb.
Helps reduce pains associated with periods as well as ameliorating excessive bleeding. This herb also plays a role in easing the changes of menopause. As an emmenagogue it stimulates proper menstrual flow if there is any resistance. Because of its astringency this herb is often used in diarrhea especially in children.

Doses - Tincture 2 to 4mls 3 times daily, 2 teaspoonful's of dried herb in tea 3 times daily.

Licorice

Actions - Expectorant, demulcent, anti-inflammatory, adrenal agent, anti-spasmodic, mild laxative.
The root part is used , possessing unique pectoral and emollient properties, it is also nutritive and slightly laxative, It contains the building blocks of hormones, has a marked effect on the endocrine system, catarrh,

gastric and peptic ulcers, abdominal colic. Its ability to soothe irritated mucous membranes and to break up phlegm and ease coughing sees licorice employed in respiratory conditions, coughing, bronchitis, and chest colds. Can be used for treating inflammatory and allergic conditions. Licorice has effects on the adrenal glands which are protective, restorative, tonic and stimulatory.

Uses - Treatment of cough, inflamed throat, pneumonia, pleurisy, TB, all catarrhal conditions, gallstones, chronic constipation.

Dose – 1 to 3mls of tincture 3 times daily.

Caution - Do not use with high blood pressure. Long term use depletes potassium which raises the blood pressure. Don't use with steroids.

Milk Thistle

Actions - Cholagogue, galactagogue, demulcent.
This herb is said to rejuvenate the liver, for problems like hepatitis it is used alone at first as it drains the liver probably by its action of stimulating the gallbladder to release bile. Used to increase milk production in mothers and for gallbladder problems. The reason I put this herb here is that it is the livers job to take used hormones out of the system and if this is not happening it can lead to a lot of confusion. So make sure your liver is functioning well.

Dose - Tablets can be brought in most health shops see dosage on packet.

Motherwort

Actions - Sedative, emmenagogue, antispasmodic, cardiac tonic, nervine, reproductive tonic.

Motherwort is considered a life giving plant, beneficial for all female disorders, a general heart tonic, delayed or suppressed menses especially where anxiety or tension are involved, relaxing tonic for aiding menopause, specific for over rapid heartbeat brought on by anxiety or tension.

Doses - Tincture 1 to 4mls 3 times daily, 1 to 2 teaspoonfuls of dry herb for tea 3 times a day.

Passion Flower

Actions - Sedative, antispasmodic, anodyne, relaxant, epilepsy, shingles, asthma, hypotensive.

A good herb for insomnia and a very effective herb for nerve pains especially in conditions like shingles. This herbs focus is more on restlessness and irritability, hysteria and anxiety and is soothing to the mentally worried and overworked it acts on nervousness especially due to unrest, agitation, worry, exhaustion and cerebral excitement. Used in the treatment of convulsions, epilepsy, tremors, hypertension, nervous breakdowns, migraines and neuralgias.

Doses - Tincture 1 to 4mls 3 times daily, 1 teaspoon of dried herb in tea 3 times daily.

Raspberry

Actions - Astringent, tonic, refrigerant, parturient.
Highly tonic and cleansing improving the condition of the organism during pregnancy ensuring speedy and strong expulsion of the foetus at birth. Raspberry leaf contains ferulic acid which is a uterine relaxant that can help relieve menstrual cramps. At the same time as it relaxes the uterus itself it stimulates the muscles that support the uterus which allows a easier menstrual flow.

As a astringent it can be used in diarrhea and leucorrhoea, it is valuable in easing mouth problems such as mouth ulcers, bleeding gums and inflammations

Doses - Tincture 2 to 4mls 3 times daily, 2 teaspoonful's of dried herb in tea 3 times daily.

Red Clover

Actions - Alterative, diuretic, eczema, expectorant, antispasmodic, bronchitis, whooping cough.
Good for treating conditions like eczema and psoriasis and other chronic skin conditions.

In the respiratory system we can use the actions of expectorant and antispasmodic to treat conditions such as bronchitis, whooping cough and maybe the eczema and asthma syndrome and as this herb seems to have a affinity for the throat we could use it for tonsillitis to. In the nervous system we can use the antispasmodic action to treat stress and nervousness along with hypertension. The alterative action of this herb helps to clean out the body and makes this herbs action on the skin very effective and it is probably this action that makes it useful in cancers especially breast and Ovary cancer. This herb is in a lot of formulas now because they extract the Isoflavones (Plant Hormones) from it and it is said to be very rich in these.

The high content of hormone in this herb was first noted by farmers in New Zealand who noticed that sheep which grazed on Red Clover became infertile.

Doses - Tincture 2 to 6mls 3 times a day. 1 to 3 teaspoon full of dried herb in tea 3 times a day.

Rosemary

Actions - Circulatory and nerve stimulant, carminative, anti-spasmodic, anti-depressive, cholagogue.

This herb acts as a circulatory and nerve stimulant and also has a calming and toning effect on the digestive system. These actions make this herb good for the treatment of flatulence, dyspepsia, headaches, migraines, epilepsy, vertigo, fainting, low blood pressure, asthma, coughs and colds. Recently this herb has been used to prevent breast cancer and it can help to regulate menstruation.

Doses - Tincture 1 to 2mls 3 times daily, 1 to 2 teaspoons full in tea 3 times a day.

Sage

Actions - Astringent, anti-septic, inflamed throat, tonsillitis, carminative, antispasmodic, gingivitis.

This is the classic remedy for inflammations of the mouth, throat and tonsils, its volatile oils soothing the mucous membranes. This herb can be used as a mouth wash in its tea form for treating bleeding gums, inflamed tongue, or generalized mouth inflammation, mouth ulcers, laryngitis, pharyngitis, tonsillitis and quinsy. For females this herb is soothing and regulating of hormonal problems in menopause including hot flushes and is used to reduce sweats.

Doses - Tincture 2 to 4mls 3 times daily, 2 teaspoons full of herb in tea 3 times daily.

St Johns Wort

Actions - Anti-inflammatory, astringent, sedative, nervine, antiviral, nervy shooting pains.

Has a sedative and pain reducing effect which gives it a place in the treatment of neuralgia, anxiety, tension and similar problems. Regarded as a herb to use where there are menopausal changes triggering irritability and anxiety. This herb is useful for minor depression and should not be used in cases of major depression.

Doses - Tincture 1 to 4mls 3 times a day, 1 to 2 teaspoons full of dried herb in tea 3 times daily.

Schizandra

Actions - Immune stimulant, adaptogen, Nervine, antioxidant, liver tonic, restorative, cerebral tonic.

This herb is mainly focused on the liver and is used for under function and damage to this organ along with other herbs such as Milk thistle. The reason Schizandra is included in the herbal section is because it also improves mental, physical and sensory performance and helps in the handling of stress and increases stamina. This herb can also help with night sweats and improve a poor memory and is good for the treatment of depression.

Dose - 1500mg to 8000mg per day.

Sarsaparilla

Actions - Alterative, diuretic, diaphoretic, demulcent, anti-rheumatic.

Has chemicals and properties that aid in the production of testosterone, eliminates poisons and toxins from the blood and helps clean the system, useful in scaling skin conditions such as psoriasis, used in rheumatism and arthritis. Can be used for PMS problems and for menopause as well especially for loss of interest in sex. Mixed with Penny Royal it can help to relieve hot flashes.

Doses - Tincture take to 2mls 3 times a day, 1 to 2 teaspoonful's of root in tea 3 times daily.

Shepherds Purse

Actions - Uterine stimulant, astringent, diuretic, urinary antiseptic.

Possesses important astringent properties as well as being a gentle diuretic. It has a specific use in the stimulation of the menstrual process while also being used to reduce excess flow or any other type of bleeding condition in the area. Organ remedy for kidneys and bladder, tonic to pelvic organs.

Doses - Tincture 1 to 2mls 3 times a day, 1 to 2 teaspoonful of dried herb in tea 3 times a day.

Skullcap

Actions - Nerve tonic, sedative, antispasmodic, stress, anxiety, PMS, antidepressive, alterative.

Skullcap has a wide range of use mostly focusing on the nerves. It relaxes states of nervous tension while at the same time renewing and revivifying the central nervous system. It has a specific use in the treatment of seizure, epilepsy and hysterical states. It may be used in all exhausted or depressed conditions. Good for easing Pre Menstrual Tension and painful menstruation.

Doses - Tincture 2 to 4mls 3 times a day, 1 to 2 teaspoonful's of dried herb in tea 3 times a day.

Squaw Vine

Actions - Astringent, nerve tonic, diuretic,

emmenagogue, restorative, dysmenorrhoea, parturient

This herb can be taken for the relief of painful periods, amenorrhea, menorrhagia, uterine bleeding and chronic congestion of the uterus. Squaw Vine is more well known for preparing the body for child birth and helping with complications after birth.

Doses - Tincture 1 to 2mls 3 times a day, 1 teaspoonful of herb in tea 3 times a day.

Valerian

Actions - Sedative, hypnotic, antispasmodic, hypotensive, anxiety, PMS, antidepressive.

One of the most relaxing nervines available that can be used to safely reduce tension and anxiety and is also a very effective herb for chronic insomnia. As a antispasmodic it will give relief to any cramp like and colicky pains and is a good pain reliever in general helping with rheumatic and migraine pains. Can also be used for nervous exhaustion and high blood pressure.

Doses - Tincture 2 to 4mls 3 times daily. 1 to 2 teaspoons full of root in tea 3 times daily.

Vervain

Actions - Nerve tonic, sedative, antispasmodic, diaphoretic, hepatic, antidepressive, hypnotic.

This herb is a combination of a Nervine and a Hepatic so it can be used to treat doth systems. As a Nervine it can be used for stress, tension and as a general relaxant and it is also used to ease depression and melancholia especially after illness or influenza. As a hepatic it has been found to be of help for problems such as inflammation of the gallbladder and jaundice. This herb may be of some help in migraine headaches.

Doses - Tincture 2 to 4mls 3 times a day. 1 to 3 teaspoonful's of dried herb in tea 3 times daily.

Vitex Agnus Castus (Chaste Tree)

Actions - Hormone balancer, progesterone precursors, PMS, menopause.

This herb has a stimulating and normalizing effect on the pituitary glands functions especially its progesterone function. The main use of this herb is for normalizing the activity of female hormones and is indicated for dysmenorrhea, PMS, Menopause and is also used to help restore balance for female going of birth control pills. Other uses are Acne and Endometriosis.

Doses - Tincture 1 to 2mls 3 times a day, 1 teaspoonful of the ripe berries in tea 3 times a day.

Note - This herb may take a month or 2 to start working and when it does start working it is necessary to take the herb for 3 to 6 months after symptoms disappear.

Yarrow

Actions - Astringent, digestive, diuretic, antiseptic, peripheral vaso dilator, menstrual regulator.

A good herb for fevers and for lowering blood pressure. As a antiseptic diuretic Yarrow is good for the treatment of cystitis and is also used to regulate menstruation at puberty and menopause.

Doses - Tincture 2 to 4mls 3 times a day. 1 to 2 teaspoonful's of dried herb for tea 3 times a day.

Wild Yam

Actions - Antispasmodic, anti-inflammatory, ovary and uterine pains, visceral relaxant, colic.

This herb was once the sole source of the chemicals that were used in the early contraceptive pill. The antispasmodic action makes it valuable for the relief of colic and menstrual cramps and dysmenorrhea along with ovarian and uterine pains. Good for nervy type pains.

Doses - Tincture 2 to 4mls 3 times a day, 1 to 2 teaspoonful's in tea 3 times a day.

Withania (Ashwagandha)

Actions - Adaptogen, analgesic, anti-tumor, hormone regulator, pregnancy tonic, rejuvinative.

This herb is a pregnancy tonic for both the foetus and a weak mother, relieves pain by lowering serotonin levels which contribute to the sensitivity of pain receptors in the body. Good for debility, nervous exhaustion especially due to stress and chronic diseases especially those marked by inflammation. Retards various aspects of the aging process and increases stamina and also sexual desire.

Doses - As on packet.

Zizyphus

This is the new kid on the block that is being used in a lot of the new menopause formulas and also sleeping remedies. This herb has been used in Chinese medicine for over 4000 years. One write up I read said. The seed is used in TCM to quieten the spirit, for dream disturbed sleep, insomnia, irritability, palpations with anxiety and spontaneous night sweats.

Homeopathic Supplement

Homeopathy has been around now for hundreds of years and unlike most other forms of medicine its rules have not changed and will not for they are based on an essential truth. The main rule is Like cures Like or if we break down the word Homeopathy homo means the same and pathy means disease. As Homoeopathy is a very hard science to learn and as it kind of sits or balances on the border of hard science and metaphysics I will not try to explain to you what it is here as it would probably take a whole book to do this but I will say this, in the UK and a lot of countries in Europe it is on and paid for by the National Health System and anything that can get a politician to open their purse must work.

It is said that Homeopathy sits on a three legged stool. What this means is that if a remedy has at least three symptoms in the same strength as the symptoms you are trying to match then that remedy is a potential cure for your condition or if not cure it will offer the condition relief. The more symptoms you can match to the remedy the better the remedy will work for the rule is likes cure likes not vaguely similar cures. Listed below are some common Homoeopathic Remedies and some of the symptoms they cover. The idea is to find one remedy that covers most of your symptoms. To make the remedies as closer a match as we can we ask lots of questions like the ones below and after we gather all the answers we have what is called a good Symptom Picture which we then try to match as accurately as we can to a Remedy. Most Homeopathic Materia Medicas are set out to answer the questions listed below with the mind symptoms being the most important. Questions on time, position and temperature are good for making a choice between to very close remedies. The best Materia Medica for the lay person is Boerickes and you should be able to view this on a few Homeopathic websites.

Symptom Questions Guide

1/. Was there a sudden onset of the condition, at what time?

2/. What time of the day does the patient feel either better or worse.

3/. What is the effect of motion? jarring? walking? running?

4/. What is the effect of drinking fluids? warm and or cold drinks?

5/. Is the patient thirsty or not at all? sips or gulps?

6/. Is the onset from exertion? overeating? weather changes? emotions?

7/. Mental emotional state of patient?

8/. Better warm room? warm air?

9/. Better cool room? cool open air?

10/. Are the respirations upper chest movements or in the abdomen?

11/. Respirations - dry or wet?

12/. Expectoration - watery or stringy mucous, easy or difficult.

13/. Is there coughing

14/. Position - better or worse from sitting? standing? lying? lying on which side?

15/. Along with the condition is there fever? gas? belching? wind?

Modality - The questions above are covering what the Homoeopaths call modalities which basically mean are covering a condition that makes the patient better or worse. I will list the main Modalities below. The Modalities help us to distinguish which remedy is right for the case especially when we have a group that look as though they may all work which is what I am giving you und the disease heading. Using modalities forces you to think what really is going on, is this the nature of the beast or the nature of the disease.

Time - Better or Worse morning, night, weekly, monthly, seasonally etc.

Motion - Better or Worse first movement, rest, exertion, walking, stretching, rising up etc

Temperature - Better or Worse heat, cold, cold air blowing, sudden change etc.

Body Activity - Better or Worse eating, drinking, urinating, defecating, sleep, coughing etc

Weather - - Better or Worse, damp, sunny, foggy, storms, sudden changes etc.

Senses - Better or Worse - touch, pressure, noise, light, odors etc.

Position - Better or Worse lying, standing, sitting, stretched out, doubled up, right side etc.

Mind - Excitement, anger, fear, stress, better busy, nervous all the time etc.

Now read through all the remedies in the Marteria Medica (Homoeopathic Remedy Reference) and you will notice that most of them have Mind or mental symptoms kind of describing the personalities or moods a good example is Nux Vomica, I think we all know a nasty type of individual that this remedy would be suited to and meaning as though the individual is suited to this remedy then the remedy would have a curative action on them but don't expect it to change the nature of the beast. One of the main rules of Homeopathy is the closer the match of the remedy the higher the Potency you use but if you are not used to Homoeopathy just use the 30C potency and remember what I said about the 3 legged stool. Potency is a measure of strength and depth of action.

Remember as mentioned before Homoeopathy sits on a three legged stool. What this means is that if a remedy has at least three symptoms in the same strength as your symptoms then that remedy is a potential cure.

Note - The best prescribing guide for the layman is **Boerickes Materia Medica With Repertory.**

Another good guide is **The Complete Book Of Homeopathy by Dr Michael Weiner.**

I always buy my books on Homeopathy from India as they are quarter the price and there is always a wide selection. Put B. Jain Publishers into the google search engine go to their web site and check out these books and I am sure you will be pleased with what you find.

Treatment Using The Kit

The kit that used to be supplied was 4 Homoeopathic Complexes based on the symptoms of the main groups of PMS. As Homoeopathy is a very hard science to learn and as it kind of sits or balances on the boarder of hard science and metaphysics I will not try to explain to you what it is here as it would probably take a whole book to do this but I will say this, in the UK and a lot of countries in Europe it is on and paid for by the National Health System and anything that can get a politician to open their purse must have a lot of truth in it.

For the kit I am not using Homoeopathy in the way it was designed but am grouping together certain remedies to cover certain groups of symptoms hence the name Complexes. Before using the kit you should be well on the way to sorting out your diet and you should be using the supplements that you feel you need for your appropriate symptoms as well as having made some good lifestyle changes especially on the exercise and de-stressing side.

The Four Complexes

1. **PMS(A).**   The complex that we will use for this has the two hormones estrogen and progesterone in it. I have made this complex in such a way that it will

reduce the strength of estrogen and encourage more production of progesterone. The other 4 remedies I have in this complex will help to counter the symptoms of anxiety, irritability, mood swings and nervous tension. **<u>Do not mix with PMS(D).</u>**

Remedies – Estrogen 9C, Progesterone 4C, Chamomile 7C, Sepia 6C, Nux Vom 6C,Kali Mur 6X.

2.   PMS(B) Mixer.   In this complex there are no hormones so you can safely mix it with another. There are 4 remedies in this complex and they will help to counter the symptoms of fluid retention, weight gain, breast tenderness, abdominal tenderness, swollen hands and feet. This complex mixes well with PMS(A) as PMS(A) has the low estrogen hormone in it and high estrogen is part of the cause for bloating.

Remedies – Nat Mur 6X, Apis 6C, Strophanthus 6C, Apocynum 6X.

3.   PMS(C) Mixer.   In this complex there are no hormones so you can safely mix it with another. There are 4 remedies in this complex and they will help to counter the symptoms of food cravings, headache, fatigue, dizziness and palpitation.

Remedies – Nat Mur 6X, Sepia 6C, Conium 7C, Cyclamen 5C.

4.   PMS(D).   This complex has the hormones estrogen and progesterone in it. The complex will encourage estrogen production and reduce the production of progesterone this is the opposite of PMS(A) so for obvious reasons do no mix with PMS(A). The other 4 remedies in this complex cover the symptoms of depression, crying, forgetfulness, confusion and insomnia.

Remedies – Estrogen 4C, Progesterone 9C, Pulsatilla 6C, Nat Mur 6X, Sepia 6C.

How to Take The Complexes

1/. The 4 bottles are your stock complexes and must not be mixed together.

2/. To take a dose place 15mls of pure water in your measurer cup and add 4 drops of the stock complex.

3/. If you wish to make a mixture of 2 or more complexes just add the stock complex needed to the water in the measuring cup. (Never mix the stock complexes together).

4/. When you have prepared what you need sip your dose slowly.

5/. Do not eat, drink, smoke or clean teeth for about 15 minutes before or after taking a remedy.

6/. Dosage is about 3 to 4 times daily.

Example Of A Dose

These complexes are designed to be to be mixed and matched to your personal symptoms so for example if you had PMS(A) with the added symptoms of fluid retention you could add PMS(B) Mixer to your dose as well. If on the next day the bloating was gone and you started to get the headaches and food cravings of PMS(C) you could change your mix accordingly. What you can never do is have a dose of PMS(A) and PMS(D) together as they will cancel themselves out as the hormones in these are opposites.

How To Use This Section

In the Marteria medica that follows you are given most of the Homoeopathic remedies that are used in the Complexes. The symptoms guide gives you the knowledge of the questions to ask to find a good Homoeopathic remedy which you can use to find with the many online repertories that are available. When you have found a remedy that you think suits you look it up in Boerickes Marteria Medica as this is one of the easiest to use even though it is in old English. The hormones I have used is a slightly different form of Homoeopathy that I kind of think of as body parts homoeopathy. Generally it works like this. A low 4C potency of Estrogen tries to stimulate the body to produce more Estrogen while a 9C potency of Estrogen makes the body think there is too much thus reducing Estrogen. This can be used for example in my PMS kit where sometimes I want to reduce a hormone as it may be leading to unwanted problems so I give it in the 9C potency with an example being Progesterone 9C to try to lower it. Now you can start to see a whole new method of controlling Hormones.

Materia Medica

Note - All Homeopathic Remedies are given in Potency and not in material Form.

Aconite

Characteristics - Aconite is best used in the first stages of a illness, especially when fear and anxiety are present. Symptoms appear suddenly, without warning and they may be caused by exposure to cold winds or draughts or by a severe fright. Symptoms are a marked restlessness, displays extreme anxiety or fear, high fever with a burning skin, extreme sweating and a burning thirst, a hoarse dry painful cough, bright light noises stress and cold worsen the symptoms, rest and quiet relieves the symptoms. The pains of Aconite are unbearable, sharp, shooting, burning pains, tingling and numbness. A remedy for fevers and inflammatory states, use at the first sign of all fevers, shivering with cold sweats, difficult breathing, shows desire for large quantities of water, symptoms worse at midnight, symptoms improve in the open air. In women dry vagina. Menses to profuse, ovaries congested and painful.

Mind - Great fear, anxiety, restlessness, extreme sensitivity to pain, worry, foreboding.

Better - In open air, warmth, rest.

Worse - In the evening and night, particularly before midnight, lying on affected side.

Allium Cepa

Characteristics - Increased secretions from the eyes and nose, like those of the common cold. Frequent sneezing with watery discharge which burns the nose and upper lip, but the eye discharge is bland and doesn't burn (the opposite of Euphrasia). Tickling in the throat with incessant cough (feels as if larynx is split) holds throat when coughing. Being in cool open air relieves the symptoms, eyelids are swollen and red, abdominal tympany with wind, this remedy is indicated in the early stages of most catarrhal conditions..

Better - Cold room (except cough), open air.

Worse - Evening, warm room, odors.

Antimonium Tartaricum - Ant Tart

Characteristics - Is characterized by a loose rattling unproductive cough.. Respiration can be very difficult with much gasping. There is usually thirst for little and often. Symptoms are worse in the evening, lying down and in cold damp weather or a warm room. Confined largely to respiratory diseases, abundant bronchial secretions, great rattling of mucous with little expectoration, drowsiness, debility and sweat. Burning in urethra during and after urinating, last drops bloody with pain in the bladder, urging increased.

Mind - Drowsy and despondent, fear of being alone, child will not be touched without whining.

Better - Sitting erect, from burping and expectoration.

Worse - Evenings, lying down, damp cold weather.

Apis

Characteristics - Apis is used for various types of swelling and inflammation such as that from animal bites and bites and stings from insects, it is also used for measles, mumps, sore throats, sore red eyes and fever. Apis is a quick acting remedy for inflammations especially those ones with edema and lots of swelling which is its main use. Acute nephritis with scanty and burning urine there may be some blood in the urine. . Symptoms are swelling with edema which makes the effected parts look shiny, red and puffy, the swollen parts feel soggy and waterlogged, a fever that develops rapidly but without thirst, extreme restlessness and fidgeting, an irritable nature and perhaps jealous, cool air and cold compresses relieve the symptoms. Pains are burning and stinging, arthritis with swelling, animals seek cold surface to lie on, swollen eyelids, may be swollen ears, may be blood in the urine. Symptoms get worse from heat and improve in the open air and from cold bathing. In women edema of the vulva, inflammation of the ovaries, stinging pains, dysmenorrhea with severe ovarian pain, ovarian tumors, metritis with stingy pains, burning and soreness when urinating, incontinence.

Mind - Apathy, indifference, awkward.

Better - By cold, (room, air or application)

Worse - From warmth, pressure, late in the afternoon, from sleeping.

Arnica

Characteristics - Bruises and similar injuries where the skin is unbroken and there is mental or emotional shock. Symptoms are any type of bruising or similar injury caused by crushing, squeezing or wrenching, muscles strains which feel sore and bruised, shock after accidents, there is a fear of being touched because of the pain, good for the soreness after birth and medical operations.

Arnica can be used in potency and also as a cream. The cream must not be used on broken skin or wounds

Mind - Fears touch or approach, whole body oversensitive.

Better - Lying down or with head low.

Worse - Least touch, motion, damp and cold.

Arsenic Album

Characteristics - Burning pains relieved by heat, anxious, restless, weak and chilly with an air of fear and hopelessness. Anxiety or restlessness are often present where this remedy is indicated. Discharge from eyes and nose are watery and acrid causing ulceration in those regions. The mouth is usually dry and the patient is usually thirsty. Dramatic vomiting and diarrhea often simultaneously indicate its use if the modalities agree. The patient may have wheezing respiration and allergic asthmatic conditions can respond well. The skin can be dry, scaly and scruffy. Symptoms are worse for cold and wet better for warmth. Tries to find relief in motion but immediately feels weak with movement. Restless, feels cold, complains of general weakness, discharges burn the skin. For women menses to profuse to soon, burning in ovarian region, leucorrhoea acrid, burning, offensive and thin, bladder as if paralyzed.

Mind - Fear with despair and restlessness.

Better - Warmth, open air, relieved by sweat, hot drinks, lying down (but restless).

Worse - Cold air, after midnight eg 1 to 3am. Wet damp weather and near sea shore.

Belladonna

Characteristics - This is one of the great fever remedies, conditions requiring its use usually being of violent and sudden onset. Heat, redness, pain and swelling characterize its symptoms. It is one of the main remedies used in convulsions. Pupils are usually dilated which is a keynote for this remedy. Acute ear inflammation where there is heat, pain and swelling respond well. The mouth is usually dry and there is great thirst. With Belladonna always think BIRDS. B for burning, I for irritability, R for redness, D for delirium and S for spasms. For women acute urinary infections, urine frequent and profuse, sensitive forcing downward, as if all the viscera would protrude at genitals, dryness and heat in vagina, menses increased bright red to early, to profuse, mastitis pain, breasts feel heavy and hard and red, tumors of breast.

Mind - Hallucinations, delirium, rages, bites, strikes, desire to escape.

Better - For quiet, dark, rest with slight warmth.

Worse - For noise, touch or jarring motion.

Bellis Perennis

Characteristics - Trauma to abdomen and pelvic organs especially after surgery and child birth if arnica does not give relief. Injuries to the nerves with intense soreness, back ache from hard physical work such as gardening, pain is bruised sore and aching, better cold presses, worse touch, after getting wet. Unwilling to move and when made to do so causes pain, muscular stiffness is prominent. In women uterus feels sore as if squeezed.

Worse - Left side and cold wind.

Bryonia

Characteristics - This remedy shows both diarrhea and constipation symptoms, the latter usually in chronic conditions. The mouth is often dry and there is great thirst. The tongue is often coated yellow. It is of great help in many cases of rheumatism or arthritis where the symptoms agree. There is often respiratory signs with a hoarse hacking cough. All symptoms are worse for movement and better for rest. In women menses to early, to profuse, worse from motion, menses suppressed with headache, ovary pains tender to touch, pain in breasts during period, breasts hot and painful, menstrual irregularities with gastric problems.

Mind - Irritable, delirium.

Better - Lying on the painful side, pressure, rest and cold things.

Worse - Warmth, motion, morning, eating and touch.

Calendula

Characteristics - The part used is the Flowers and it is used for wounds and skin irritations, it is healing, soothing, anti-inflammatory, astringent, anti-fungal and anti-microbial.

Use as a lotion for cuts, grazes, infected sores, fungal infections, any skin inflammations, regulates the oil production of the skin so is good for acne, to stop bleeding, for bruises and sprains, skin ulcers and minor burns and scolds.

Note - The tincture of this is used as a lotion diluted at 1 to 10.

Cantharis

Characteristics - Important first aid remedy for minor burns and for other pains that feel burning and fiery, also has a healing effect on the bladder, urethra and other parts of the urinary tract where burning pain is the key symptom, burns and scalds especially where blistering and inflammation occur, sunburn, insect bites that feel hot and burn, cystitis. Pains are violent burning, cutting, stabbing or smarting, rawness.

Mind - Furious delirium, acute mania generally of a sexual type, crying, barking.

Better - Better from warmth rest and rubbing.

Worse - From touch or approach, from urinating, from drinking cold water.

Carbo Vegetabilis

Characteristics - Patient exhibits mental and physical sluggishness and symptoms come on slowly, generalized weakness of all functions especially digestion, overweight, torpid, lazy, complaints of coldness, pains usually described as burning, pressing pains, wishes to be fanned, digestive problems such as belching often accompany any illness. In women menses copious an early, swollen vulva leucorrhoea before menses thick greenish milky and excoriating, during menses burning in hands and soles.

Mind - Aversion to darkness, sudden loss of memory.

Better - Being fanned, passing gas, rest.

Worse - Morning and evening, exertion, cold, tight clothes at abdomen.

Causticum

Characteristics - Burns and burning pains such as cystitis also used for dry coughs, burns to the skin especially with marked inflammation and blistering, coughs, laryngitis and hoarseness from straining and over using voice, cystitis especially with involuntary passing of urine when coughing, chronic cystitis, exposure to cold dry air may make symptoms worse. For women menses cease at night only flows during day.

Mind - Least thing makes it cry, sad, hopeless. Ailments from long lasting grief.

Better - In damp wet weather, warmth.

Worse - Cold winds.

Cimicfuga

Characteristics – This remedy has a wide action on the nerves and muscles. Nervous subjects with ovarian irritation and nervy pain, uterine cramps and heavy limbs. Agitation and pain indicate this remedy, pains like electric shocks here and there. Migraine symptoms. Amenorrhea, pain immediately before menses, menses always irregular. Ovarian pains, Oversensitive to pain.

Mind – Great depression and low spirits,, incessant talking.

Better – Warmth and eating

Worse – Morning, cold, during menses.

Euphrasia

Characteristics - Affects the mucous membranes of the eyes, nose and chest producing copious watery secretions, eye secretions cause smarting of the skin while the nose discharge is bland. Used for conjunctivitis, eye strain generally but especially from computers, eyes that feel sore and inflamed and look red, hay fever symptoms including a tickly throat, sneezing, a runny nose, and itchy red watering eyes. Sunlight wind and warmth worsen the symptoms. In women menses painful, flow lasts only an hour or day, amenorrhea with ophthalmia.

Better - In the dark

Worse - From light, indoors, in the evening.

Hypericum

Characteristics - Used for bruises and other injuries especially to nerve rich areas like the fingers, lips, ears, eyes ,tail bone, good for the pain of puncture wounds of any cause eg animal or insect. Helps with the pains after operations especially amputations. Pains are violent shooting pains along a nerve path, burning, tingling and numbness. Worse from shock and touch and better from rubbing, horse fly bites, symptoms worse cold better warmth.

Mind - Anxiety, melancholy, effects of shock.

Better - Bending head backward.

Worse - Cold, dampness and touch.

Ignatia

Characteristics – Suited for the nervous. sensitive, highly conscientious, excitable people with gentle dispositions. The emotional state is of quick alternating moods. Labor like pains. Menses to profuse or scanty. Feminine sexual frigidity.

Mind – Changeable moods, introspective, silently brooding, melancholic, sad, tearful. Not commutative.

Better – Change of position, hard pressure.

Worse – Morning. Coffee, external warmth.

Ipecac

Characteristics - Indicated for complaints of persistent nausea not relieved by vomiting, ailments caused by eating rich or indigestible type of foods such as ice-cream, sweets etc., useful to stop bleeding if blood is bright red. For women uterine hemorrhage profuse bright blood gushing with nausea, pain from navel to uterus.

Mind - Easily irritated, child cries or screams continuously, wanting something but not sure what they desire, holds everything in contempt.

Worse - Warm, moist weather, lying down.

Kali Bichromicum

Characteristics - Has an affinity for the mucous membranes of the body, tough stringy viscid secretions sometimes forming thick yellow green mucous, sinus infections, suited for fleshy fat light complexioned people, general weakness.

Better - Heat

Worse - Cold, beer, morning, undressing.

Kali Carbonicum

Characteristics - Has an affinity for the mucous membranes digestive and respiratory, very tired, anemic, flabby tissues which may be swollen, sweat, backache, weakness, many conditions have an aggravation at 2am to 4am, often stays immobile when ill.For women menses early, profuse or to late pale and scanty.

Mind - Very irritable, hypersensitive to pain, despondent.

Better - During the day, sitting down, bending forward, warmth.

Worse - Cold weather, between 2am and 4am.

Lachesis

Characteristics - Many symptoms tend to be left sided, cannot bear tight clothing, symptoms worse on awakening, symptoms relieved with onset of the menstrual flow. Short dry cough, feels relief after coughing up watery phlegm, feeling of constriction in throat and chest, better bending forward. For women climacteric troubles, palpitations, flashes of heat, menses to short to feeble, all pains relieve by the flow, left ovary painful and swollen.

Mind - Overly talkative, impatient, sad, jealous, no desire to mix with world.

Better - Release of pressure, eating fruit, cold, discharges.

Worse - Pressure, touch, after sleep, heat, hot weather.

Ledum

Characteristics - Has an action on the capillaries and is useful for cleaning up bruises especially around the eyes, mainly used for puncture wounds made by sharp points such as nails and wood splinters and insect bites and stings especially ones that don't heal properly and look blue and puffy. Wounds that feel cold to the touch, septic conditions, sprains, pains are throbbing, tearing ,prickling, they shoot upwards, stiff and sore. Better cold, cold bathing. This remedy was used in the past along with hypericum to ward off tetanus especially in deep wounds

Better - From cold.

Worse - At night and from heat.

Lycopodium

Characteristics - Exerts most of its effects on the digestive organs, liver, kidneys and respiratory systems. The patient dislikes being left alone and appears apprehensive. The nose is often blocked and there may be blisters on the tongue. Eating a little food always satisfies the appetite but appetite is very marked. The belly is usually bloated. The stool appears hard and small and is expelled only with difficulty accompanied by ineffectual straining. Urination is also a slow process and the urine has a red sediment. For women vagina dry, sex painful, right ovarian pain, leucorrhoea acrid with burning in the vagina.

Mind - Melancholy, afraid to be alone, apprehensive.

Better - By motion, on getting cold.

Worse - From heat.

Natrum Sulphuricum

Characteristics - A good liver remedy, emotional and mental difficulties arising after head injury, useful in problems associated with rainy weather and dampness, patient feels every change from dry to wet weather, may remove excess water and fluid retention from the body. For women menses irregular, usually profuse, vagina dry, leucorrhoea acrid and watery.

Mind - Lively music saddens, melancholy, inability to think, dislikes to speak or be spoken to.

Better - Dry weather and environments, pressure, change of position.

Worse - Damp weather, damp basements, lying on left side.

Nux Vom

Characteristics - The remedy for overindulgence, adapted especially to thin irritable energetic people who attend with great detail to tasks, quarrelsome, nervous, intelligent, hypochondriacal, oversensitive to noise music and light, craves stimulants.

Primarily used in the digestive sphere, its greatest reputation is in helping disturbances following overeating of unsuitable foods. Feces is usually hard but diarrhea can follow overeating. There is abdominal discomfort, flatulence, irritability and sensitivity to noise. For women menses to early lasts to long, always irregular, prolapse.

Mind - Very irritable, sensitive to all impressions, malicious, disposed to reproach others.

Better - Wet weather, lying down, uninterrupted nap.

Worse - Overeating, mental over exertion, sensory stimulation ie sound, sight, touch etc.

Phosphorus

Characteristics - Irritated and inflamed mucous and serous membranes are the key feature of this remedy. Is a very sudden remedy with suddenness of symptoms. The patient is sensitive to loud and sudden noises (eg thunder fireworks etc). Degenerative processes and bone destruction respond well to Phosphorus. Food is suddenly vomited back up when it has been warmed in the stomach, gums can be ulcerated and bloody. Hepatitis, jaundice, pancreatic disease and nephritis come into its sphere. Urine may be bloody. A very painful cough is also a symptom. Wounds that perpetually bleed may also be helped. The patient is usually in poor body condition. For women menses to early and scanty, lasts to long, leucorrhoea profuse, smarting, corrosive, instead of menses.

Mind - Low spirits, restless, fidgety.

Better - In the dark, lying on the right side, from the cold, sleep.

Worse - Touch, from exertion and in the evening.

Pulsatilla

Characteristics - Often indicated for those with mild, gentle, timid yielding dispositions who are easily moved to laughter and tears, The Pulsatilla person wants to be held and loved, moods changeable and fickle, the patient is chilly but desires strolling in cold air, symptoms are erratic and change frequently, pains are wandering, pains that grow gradually in intensity, fever without thirst despite dry mouth, bland yellow discharges. Changeable menstrual flow, starting and stopping.

Mind - Weeps easily, timid, fears to be alone - dark - ghosts, likes sympathy and fuss, highly emotional, easily discouraged, sensitive.

Better - Open air, cold applications, consolation relieves symptoms.

Worse - Evening before midnight, warmth, after eating fat rich food.

Rhus Tox

Characteristics - Is the most famous of the rheumatic remedies. The skin and muscular skeletal system are its main spheres. Small red papules in the skin and sometimes vesicles are typical lesions with much scratching. In all cases of damage to muscles think of Rhus and the symptoms of arthritis which are worse after rest particularly if this follows strenuous exertion. The symptoms improve with limbering up , The worst pains are seen as the animal arises from its bed. For women swelling with intense itching of vulva, menses early, profuse and prolomged, acrid.

Mind - Listless, sad, extreme restlessness, great apprehension at night.

Better - Warmth, walking, from stretching out limbs.

Worse - During sleep, cold wet rainy weather and at night.

Ruta

Characteristics - Has effects on the joints, tendons, cartilages, and the periosteum which is a fine membrane that covers bones and gives it that shiny look, it is also used for eye strain where the vision goes dim.

Used for painful bruises affecting the bones, dislocations, strains to the tendons or joints, aching with restlessness, pains are gnawing, digging, burning, bruised, sore as if beaten, bones as if broken, pain deep in the bones, rheumatism.

Better - From lying and warmth.

Worse - From over exertion, touch, cold wet weather.

Silica

Characteristics - Fits the shy chilly patient who is reluctant to enter the room, chronic inflammatory conditions such as sinus, helps in the removal of foreign bodies such as splinters and seeds, ripens abscesses, ailments attended with pus formation. Use silica and be prepared to use it for a while sometimes up to 3 weeks. For women leucorrhoea milky acrid, itching of vulva and vagina, discharge of blood between periods, vaginal cysts.

Mind - Faint hearted, anxious, yielding.

Better - Warmth, wet or humid weather.

Worse - Morning, from lying down, cold.

Staphysagria

Characteristics - Suits sensitive people who suppress their feelings and suffer in silence or who boil over with indignation, remedy for cuts and wounds especially those that are from medical procedures and have the mentioned feelings. Nervous states of animals. The pains are stinging, stitching, smarting, squeezing, as if stabbed by a knife. Worse from touch, emotions and suppressed anger. For women part very sensitive, worse sitting down, prolapse.

Better - Warmth, rest at night.

Worse - Touch on affected parts, loss of fluids.

Sepia

Characteristics – Often pale flabby persons with fair but flushed skin, sensitive to external influences such as touch and jarring. Exhausted dragging down sensations, better in the afternoon, wore in the morning and evening. Ailments from sexual excess. prone to problems of the sexual organs. Organs feel as if forced out through vulva, menses usually late and scant. Leucorrhoea yellow, greenish with much itching, menses to late, scanty, irregular, prolapse, vagina painful especially during sex.

Mind – Indifferent to those loved best, averse to occupation, to family. Dreads to be alone. Very sad. Weeps when telling symptoms.

Better – Afternoon and from exercise.

Worse – Morning, evening, sensory stimuli such as touch, light, noise and storms.

Symphytum

Characteristics - Causes bone to grow and promotes fast healing should be given for all fractures. Used for injuries to the hard parts of the body while arnica is for the soft parts. Also used for eye injuries caused from blows.

Caution - do not use if a pin has been placed in the bone as the pin has to be removed latter.

Tarentula Cubensis

Characteristics - For abscesses, boils, carbuncles, swellings of any kind but especially on the back of the neck where the skin turns black, red/blue or purple with great pain. Deep septic conditions with hardening of the effected part, condition comes on fast, pains are burning, stinging, throbbing, pricking like a needle.

Worse - Night.

Urtica Urens

Characteristics - Can be used for burns and also for cystitis where the urine burns the skin and there is difficulty passing urine. Symptoms are stinging pains, swellings particularly blistery swellings, itching. For women leucorrhoea acid and excoriating, uterine hemorrhage, stinging and itching of the vulva with odema, excessive swelling of the breasts.

Worse - Cool moist air, touch

Disclaimer

The information in this booklet is given as a General Guide and the author accepts no responsibility for self-treatment and advices that if you are in doubt seek Professional Help.